100   swers
About HIV and AIDS
THIRD EDITION

Joel Gallant, MD, MPH

Medical Director of Specialty Services
Southwest CARE Center
Santa Fe, New Mexico

JONES & BARTLETT
LEARNING

World Headquarters
Jones & Bartlett Learning
5 Wall Street
Burlington, MA 01803
978-443-5000
info@jblearning.com
www.jblearning.com

Jones & Bartlett Learning books and products are available through most bookstores and online booksellers. To contact Jones & Bartlett Learning directly, call 800-832-0034, fax 978-443-8000, or visit our website, www.jblearning.com.

Substantial discounts on bulk quantities of Jones & Bartlett Learning publications are available to corporations, professional associations, and other qualified organizations. For details and specific discount information, contact the special sales department at Jones & Bartlett Learning via the above contact information or send an email to specialsales@jblearning.com.

Production Credits

Executive Acquisitions Editor: Nancy Anastasi Duffy
Editorial Assistant: Jade Freeman
Associate Production Editor: Alex Schab
Manufacturing and Inventory Control Supervisor: Amy Bacus
Marketing Manager: Jennifer Sharp
Composition: Miranda Design Studio, Inc.

Cover Design: Kristin E. Parker
Rights and Media Research Coordinator: Laura Piasio
Cover Images: Top left: © Photodisc
Top right: © Photos.com
Bottom: © BestPhotoStudio/ShutterStock, Inc.
Printing and Binding: Edwards Brothers Malloy
Cover Printing: Edwards Brothers Malloy

Library of Congress Cataloging-in-Publication Data

Gallant, Joel E.
  100 questions and answers about HIV and AIDS / Joel Gallant. — Third edition.
    pages cm
  ISBN 978-1-284-08986-8
  1. AIDS (Disease)—Miscellanea. 2. AIDS (Disease)—Popular works. 3. HIV infections—Miscellanea.
  4. HIV infections—Popular works. I. Title. II. Title: One hundred questions and answers about HIV and AIDS.
  RC606.64.G35 2016
  362.19697'92—dc23
                          2015016675

6048

Printed in the United States of America
19 18 17 16 15   10 9 8 7 6 5 4 3 2 1

This book is dedicated to Joel Meneses, my husband, partner, and friend, who continues to make my life richer and more joyful (even now, after three editions!).

PUBLISHER'S NOTE

The author and publisher would like to gratefully acknowledge the contribution of Mike Willis and Rose Ramroop, two patients with HIV infection who have generously shared their experience, insights, and coping tips. Throughout this book, Mike and Rose's comments provide what we hope and expect will be valuable "insider" information for readers from two individuals who are living successfully with HIV infection. Thank you, Mike and Rose.

Mike Willis lives and works in Baltimore, Maryland. He is an advocate for people with HIV disease at Chase-Brexton Health Services and is a musician in his spare time. His medication credo is: "If you can't adhere, at least comply!"

Rose Ramroop also lives in Baltimore. She has worked at Johns Hopkins University for 22 years and is now an HIV Counselor for the Johns Hopkins Women's HIV Program. She has served on the Baltimore Ryan White Planning Council and is a member of the advisory board for the Antiretroviral Pregnancy Registry. She has spoken nationally and internationally about HIV in women and children. She is the proud mother of four beautiful girls and spends her free time enjoying life with her family.

CONTENTS

CONTENTS

It is very difficult to live among people you love and hold back from offering them advice.

—Anne Tyler, *Celestial Navigation*, 1974

More than 30 years into the HIV epidemic, there is an enormous amount of information available for both patients and clinicians on HIV and AIDS. With websites and textbooks and pamphlets galore, one would wonder if there is a need for another book about AIDS. I would argue that now, more than ever, we need to help our patients take the time to ask and find answers to all of their questions about preventing and living with HIV. In this era of managed care and 15-minute medical visits, there is never enough time to do justice to all of the questions that anyone diagnosed with HIV needs to be asking. *100 Questions & Answers about HIV and AIDS* is a tremendous resource for people living with HIV, their friends, family members, and for healthcare providers. Joel Gallant, a thoughtful and seasoned HIV care provider who has been on the frontlines of HIV care for nearly two decades, has done a wonderful job framing the questions that arise from the moment of an HIV diagnosis through the many aspects of living a full life with HIV. Joel's practical, concise, and supportive answers to a wide range of questions help guide the reader through the process of adapting to an HIV diagnosis, getting into care, and making informed decisions for years to come.

Judith Currier, MD
Professor of Medicine
Chief, Division of Infectious Diseases
Associate Director, UCLA Center for
Clinical AIDS Research and Education
David Geffen School of Medicine at
University of California, Los Angeles

Introduction and Preface to the First Edition

I've been working in the field of HIV/AIDS since the beginning of the epidemic, having started my medical education at "Ground Zero"—San Francisco in 1981. My story will seem like ancient history to those of you who are too young to remember a time without AIDS, but we need history to teach us where we've been and how far we've come. My first patient on my first medical rotation as a student at San Francisco General Hospital was a terrified young gay man with *Pneumocystis* pneumonia whom I admitted to the world's first AIDS ward on the day it opened. As a terrified young gay man myself, I didn't appreciate the historical significance of that day—I was too preoccupied by my own fear. I had come out in the late 1970s, when we thought the worst thing you could get from sex was herpes, and condoms were weird things that straight guys wore to keep women from getting pregnant. I knew I was at high risk for the same disease that was killing the men I admitted to the ward. In each young man I cared for, I saw myself and my future, making it hard to appreciate the intellectual challenges or historical significance of what I was learning and experiencing.

At that time in my life, I couldn't face the thought of a medical career devoted to caring for dying gay men. In a naïve attempt to escape the plague, I left San Francisco in 1985 and moved to New Haven, Connecticut to do my medical internship and residency at Yale. I hadn't escaped, of course, but in New Haven I saw a very different epidemic, one affecting not only gay men but also drug users, heterosexual women, and their children.

There were small glimmers of hope during that time: the mid- to late-1980s. HIV was discovered as the cause of AIDS, and a blood test became available. AZT, which prevented death in early studies, was quickly approved. But AIDS remained a devastating, fatal disease that continued to expand its reach both within the United States and throughout the world. During my residency, I spent time working in hospitals in Haiti and sub-Saharan Africa. HIV testing wasn't available there at the time, but the virus made its presence felt in every clinic and on every hospital ward.

At some point during my residency, I realized that the reality of being HIV-positive couldn't be much worse than the anxiety and insomnia I was experiencing by not knowing my status. When I finally tested negative, after so many years of fear and uncertainty, things suddenly looked different. Now I could take care of people with HIV without being forced to confront my own mortality every day. Although there were detours along the way, I ultimately ended up at Johns Hopkins University, where I've been treating people with HIV infection, teaching other clinicians about HIV treatment, and doing research on HIV therapy.

In the mid-1990s, HIV infection was quickly transformed from a progressive, almost universally fatal illness to the chronic, manageable disease that it is today. The speed at which this transformation took place is unprecedented in medical history. However, HIV infection is still a serious, life-altering, and sometimes life-threatening disease.

HIV infection is unique among medical diseases. It's sexually transmitted, has caused the world's largest global epidemic, appeared only in the late 20th century, affects people who are marginalized or discriminated against, carries enormous social stigma, and has completely transformed the world we live in. This book deals primarily with medical issues, but it's impossible to discuss HIV without also talking about relationships, sex and sexuality, mental health, substance abuse, politics, and even about our place in the world and our responsibility to our fellow human beings. Whether we're dealing with HIV infection as patients, clinicians, researchers, or policymakers, we must always view HIV as both a disease that affects individuals and as an pandemic that affects societies.

ACT-UP coined the phrase "Knowledge = Power." In my experience, the people who have the most power over their disease are the ones who educate themselves, seek out expert medical care, adhere to therapy, and optimize the other aspects of their health. *100 Questions & Answers About HIV and AIDS* is not the definitive book on the subject by any means—there are other books and resources that provide more in-depth and detailed information. Instead, I hope it will serve as a starting point for people with HIV infection and for those who care about them—one that answers the questions that my own patients ask me, in language that's easy to understand. I hope this book will be the beginning of a long educational journey and that it will help you move from a position of fear to one of knowledge and power.

Joel Gallant, MD, MPH
Baltimore, Maryland
2008

Preface to the Second Edition

Because of the rapid pace of research and drug development, books about HIV infection can quickly become dated. Much has changed since the first edition of *100 Questions & Answers About HIV and AIDS* was published in 2008. The second edition has been extensively updated to include the following important developments:

- New guidelines and research supporting earlier treatment of HIV infection

- Evidence that untreated HIV infection causes inflammation and immune activation with potential long-term consequences that may include "premature aging"

- Research showing the importance of treating HIV-positive people to prevent transmission, as well as the use of pre-exposure prophylaxis (PrEP) and microbicides by HIV-negative people to prevent infection

- New drugs for the treatment of HIV infection, including new single-tablet, once-daily regimens, with updated recommendations for first-line therapy and a new table on advantages and disadvantages of the common initial regimens

- New treatments for hepatitis C coinfection that increase the possibility of cure

- Information on use of the newer vaccines (chickenpox, shingles, HPV) in HIV-positive people

- Updated recommendations on screening for osteoporosis in HIV-positive people

- The impact of changing healthcare economics, including healthcare reform, on HIV care in the United States
- Renewed optimism about someday finding a cure for HIV infection

There are many other updates and revisions that I haven't listed here, especially in the area of antiretroviral therapy. I hope that the second edition of *100 Questions & Answers About HIV and AIDS* will be informative and useful, both to seasoned readers of the first edition and to those just beginning their education.

Joel Gallant, MD, MPH
Baltimore, Maryland
2012

Preface to the Third Edition

Since the publication of the second edition of *100 Questions & Answers About HIV and AIDS,* much has changed in the world of HIV treatment and prevention—and in my own life. In 2013, after 24 years in Baltimore and 21 years on the faculty at Johns Hopkins University, my husband and I moved to Santa Fe, New Mexico, where I took a position working with my good friend Dr. Trevor Hawkins as medical director of the HIV clinic at Southwest CARE Center, a nonprofit, community-based clinic that also provides primary care and treatment for hepatitis C. Santa Fe had been my second home since the late 1990s, and as much as I loved Baltimore and my work and colleagues at Hopkins, I longed to live in the Southwest. When the position in Santa Fe became available, it felt like the perfect time to start a new phase in my life and my career. My friends and colleagues quickly divided themselves into two camps: those who thought I was crazy to leave a full professorship at Hopkins, and those were envious of my new lifestyle.

Life is good in Santa Fe, a beautiful town with the cultural and culinary richness of a big city, 300 sunny days a year, and weather that allows outdoor living 9 months out of 12. My clinic is a 15-minute bike ride from home, and beautiful mountain trails and ski slopes are just a few miles away. Our clinic is a comfortable, friendly place, full of compassionate, dedicated, and knowledgeable people, and where I can do clinical research without the bureaucratic obstacles of an academic medical center. While I sometimes miss the breadth and depth of science and medicine in an academic environment, I don't miss the constant struggle to find grant support to maintain my salary. Faculty appointments at Hopkins and the University of New Mexico let me continue teaching, and I'm still active on guidelines committees, HIV advocacy activities, and medical education. In short, I have no regrets. No one should do the same thing forever.

But enough about me. I'm not updating this book just to tell you about my move to New Mexico; there's plenty of news in the world of HIV that made a revision critical:

- Consensus, at least in the United States, that HIV therapy should be started at the time of diagnosis
- Growing evidence that there are long-term consequences of untreated HIV infection caused by chronic inflammation and immune activation
- Overwhelming support for the prevention benefits of HIV therapy
- Convincing studies showing that pre-exposure prophylaxis (PrEP) prevents HIV infection, and new U.S. guidelines supporting its use
- Improvements in HIV testing, including availability of new rapid tests and home tests, as well as fourth-generation tests that become positive sooner after infection
- New drugs for the treatment of HIV infection, including more combination tablets and single-tablet, once-daily regimens
- The availability of a new resistance test that can be performed with an undetectable viral load and can detect resistance mutations you have accumulated in the past

- Growing enthusiasm for the class of HIV drugs known as integrase inhibitors, which may now be the best choices for initial therapy in most HIV-positive people
- Revolutionary developments in the treatment and cure of hepatitis C, with approval of safe, well-tolerated, convenient treatments that can eradicate the disease in just 8–12 weeks
- The continued impact of changing healthcare economics, including healthcare reform, on HIV care in the United States
- Continued optimism—and some setbacks—in the search for an HIV cure

I hope the third edition of *100 Questions & Answers About HIV and AIDS* will be informative and useful, both to readers of the first two editions and to those just beginning their education.

Joel Gallant, MD, MPH
Santa Fe, New Mexico
2015

ACKNOWLEDGMENTS

I am indebted to many colleagues and friends, including Jean Anderson, Adriana Andrade, Michael Becketts, Todd Brown, Joseph Cofrancesco, Jeanne Marrazzo, George Siberry, and Wenoah Veikley, who reviewed sections of this book, provided valuable feedback, and found important errors. I am especially grateful to Roy Gulick, Jo Leslie, Michael Willis, and to my mother, Donna Gallant, each of whom reviewed the entire manuscript and offered invaluable suggestions. Mary Beth Hansen's comprehensive critique of the manuscript ultimately made this a far better and more useful book. Finally, I thank my patients, who teach me something new every day.

PART ONE

Now That You Know

What's my prognosis?

Can I live a normal life?
What about sex and relationships?

Who should I tell?

More...

1. What's my prognosis?

Your prognosis is excellent! HIV infection is not the progressive, fatal illness it was in the 1980s and early 1990s. The memory of those horrible times, together with the stigma that still surrounds HIV infection, can make learning you're HIV positive a lot harder than it has to be. With the right treatment, HIV infection is a chronic, manageable disease. If it didn't come with so much emotional, social, and historical baggage, people would react to the diagnosis the way they might if they learned that they had diabetes or arthritis. Granted, these aren't perfect examples, because you can't transmit diabetes or arthritis to others. On the other hand, treatment for HIV is far easier and more effective than treatment for either of those diseases.

Antiretroviral therapy (ART) is the term we use to describe the medications that stop the **virus** from replicating (multiplying or reproducing). When I speak of "therapy" in this book, I'm referring to ART. Other terms you'll sometimes hear are **highly active antiretroviral therapy** (HAART), **combination antiretroviral therapy** (cART), and the "**cocktail**," terms coined to distinguish combination therapy from the less effective treatment we used in the 1980s and early 1990s. However, since *all* ART is now HAART and cART, I find easier just to use the term "ART." By stopping the **replication** of HIV, ART keeps the **immune system**—the system in the body that fights infections and cancers—from being damaged and allows it to recover. The development of ART is up there with the discovery of antibiotics as one of the greatest medical achievements of the 20th century, and treatment keeps getting better in the 21st.

Antiretroviral therapy (ART)

Drug therapy that stops HIV from replicating and improves the function of the immune system.

Virus

A microscopic organism composed of genetic material (DNA or RNA) inside a protein coat.

Highly active antiretroviral therapy (HAART)

Antiretroviral therapy meant to suppress the viral load to undetectable levels, using a combination of several agents to prevent resistance (now usually just referred to as antiretroviral therapy [ART]).

Combination antiretroviral therapy (cART)

Another term for "HAART."

Cocktail

An outdated term for an antiretroviral regimen (a combination of antiretroviral drugs).

ART has completely changed the outlook for people with HIV infection. There is no time limit to the benefits of therapy once you start. If you take your medications faithfully, you can keep HIV in control for life—a *long* life—having to change therapy only because of side effects or because better drugs come along.

If you've just been diagnosed, plan on sticking around for a long time, living long enough to die of old age. There is no need to change your life plans based on this diagnosis.

If you start ART early and take it faithfully, you can probably live out a normal lifespan and die of old age. While we can't yet promise that the quality of your life will be exactly the same as it would have been if you weren't positive, I feel comfortable telling my patients that we can virtually eliminate the possibility that they'll ever die of AIDS.

Rose's comment:

When I was first diagnosed, I thought my life was over, and I would never live to see my kids grow up. I became self-destructive because I thought I had no future. I knew nothing about HIV except what I heard from people in the community. In the news, I heard about people facing discrimination and stigma and struggling to stay alive. I assumed that that's how life was going to be for me.

It took 8 years before I was ready to learn about the disease. I also had to learn to respect myself, rather than accepting the image that people in the community had of people like me. I live a normal life now. I work, and I have a wonderful family. I'm open now about my HIV status, and I help other HIV-positive people as a peer counselor.

Replication

The reproduction or multiplication of an organism, including HIV. The replication of HIV is a complex, multi-step process involving infection of a human cell and use of both viral enzymes and human cellular machinery to create new virus particles, which are then released and can infect new cells.

Immune system

The system in the body that fights infection.

NOW THAT YOU KNOW

If you start ART early and take it faithfully, you can probably live out a normal lifespan and die of old age.

2. Can I live a normal life? What about sex and relationships?

You *can* have a normal life...with a few adjustments. Compared to someone with no chronic medical conditions, you'll have more medical visits and will take medications. However, treatment for HIV infection is now quite simple. Many of my patients now take just one pill once a day and see me for 30 minutes every 3–6 months. They're busy with work or school, are able to travel, to stay physically active, and to maintain relationships.

The biggest adjustments are often the ones that have to do with your relationships with others. Friends and family members may have to be educated before they can treat you like they did before. Sexual relationships present a special challenge. Current partners, if they're negative, will have to face their own fear of infection— a fear not all relationships survive. Entering into new relationships involves the complex issues of **disclosure** and the fear of rejection or loss of confidentiality (Question 4).

Disclosure

The process of revealing your HIV status to others.

It may be hard to believe now, but in time, HIV infection will be low on your list of daily concerns, having little impact on the life you lead and the decisions you make. Getting to that point takes time, support, and sometimes counseling. You may feel overwhelmed now, but stick with it... *it gets better!*

3. What do I do now?

At a time like this, the last thing you may think you need is a list of tasks, but there are some important things you should do sooner rather than later. Keeping busy with constructive activities can help you cope with your new diagnosis.

- Notify your contacts: Anyone you might have infected, or who might have infected you, should be notified immediately (Questions 4 and 85).

- Find an experienced HIV healthcare provider. Question 18 discusses how to find a provider who has expertise in treating HIV infection.

- Get some lab tests. The most important tests are the **CD4 count** (or **CD4 cell count**, sometimes called "T-cell count"), **viral load (plasma HIV RNA)**, and a **resistance test**, discussed in Part 5.

- Educate yourself. Reading this book is a good start, but don't stop here. You'll find more sources of information in the Appendix.

- Think about money. How are you going to pay for care? Do you have insurance? What does it cover? Do you qualify for any benefits on the basis of your HIV infection? If you're not sure, talk to a social worker or case manager (Question 21).

- Get support. Seek out the people in your life who you can talk to about your HIV infection, and tell them. If there aren't any, find a good counselor, therapist, or support group. Don't go through this alone (Question 4)!

NOW THAT YOU KNOW

CD4 count (or CD4 cell count)

A lab test that measures the number of CD4 cells in the blood (expressed as number of cells per cubic millimeter). The CD4 count is the most important measure of immunosuppression and is the most important indicator of the need for treatment.

Viral load (or plasma HIV RNA)

A lab test that measures the amount of HIV virus in the plasma (blood), expressed as "copies per milliliter." The viral load predicts the rate of progression to AIDS. It is the most important test for measuring the effectiveness of ART and also helps determine the need for treatment.

Resistance test

A blood test (either a genotype or phenotype) that looks for HIV that is resistant to antiretroviral medications.

Mike's comment:

After my positive HIV test result, I saw a psychologist. I talked with him for a year before I got up the nerve to tell my family. Now that they know, we get along better, and I see them more often than I did before I was diagnosed. Therapy helped me to become more comfortable with myself. Facing a life-threatening illness brought up all the insecurities I'd ever felt about anything, and having someone outside of my daily life to talk to helped a lot. As my best friend said, "This way you won't run off all your friends."

4. Who should I tell?

Telling people about your HIV status is a big step, especially when you've just found out you're positive. Some people should be told right away, but with others you have time to think it over.

It's important to tell people you might have infected or who might have infected you—sex partners or people you've shared needles with. They need to find out so they can get tested, for their own benefit and to protect others. Your provider, counselor, or case manager may also be able to help you inform partners. If those don't seem like good options, state health departments can notify your contacts and advise them to get tested without revealing your name.

Think about telling friends or family members you rely on for emotional support. It's critical to have a solid support system. Think about the important people in your life. Will they be there for you? Will they respect your confidentiality? If so, consider telling them. Family members don't need to know just because they're family members. You pose no risk to them, and you may outlive them anyway. You should tell them if they'll be part of your support network.

If you're not comfortable telling friends or family members, then you need to look elsewhere. Ask about support groups, counselors, peer advocates, or therapists in your community. Internet chat groups can be lousy sources of reliable medical information, but they can be helpful places to share your experiences with other HIV-positive people in an anonymous setting.

You should also inform your healthcare providers, including doctors, dentists, counselors, and therapists. They need to know your HIV status to be able to take care of you properly. If you have a provider you don't feel you can tell, then it may be time to change providers.

You *don't* have to tell your boss, your coworkers, your plumber, or the guy sitting next to you on the bus.

There's one more issue, which I hate to mention because it makes me furious, but it's important. Many states and some cities have partner notification laws that require you to disclose your HIV status to your sex or needle-sharing partners. Failure to disclose is a crime, even if you're using a condom and no transmission occurs. HIV criminalization laws are never based on accurate science, and from a prevention standpoint they're counterproductive since they may keep people from being tested or from seeking medical care. But until we're able to get them repealed, it's important to know the laws that apply where you live.

Mike's comment:

Sometimes I had to console the people I chose to tell. I found myself having to take on the supportive role, rather than feeling supported. I also found that no one kept my secret. Be prepared.

Rose's comment:

Be careful who you tell, and tell them carefully. When I was first diagnosed 20 years ago, I told my mother and my youngest sister. They gave me a lot of support in the beginning, but they were afraid to let anyone else find out. My sister told people I would be dead from a brain tumor in 6 months. My mom would only invite me and my kids over when no one else was around. We had to drink out of paper cups, eat off paper plates, and take out our own garbage. When I didn't die in 6 months, my sister starting telling people that my daughter and I were positive, thinking she was protecting the community.

Things got better for me when I started speaking publicly about HIV. I talked about the discrimination I faced within my own family. As my family got educated, they became more supportive. They apologized for the way they had treated me, but I still felt angry.

I wound up taking care of my mother when she got cancer. I didn't show my anger because she was dying and I loved her. I wish I'd been treated the same way.

5. Should I keep working?

Most people with HIV continue to work. You've got a long life ahead of you, and you're going to need the money and insurance, not to mention the opportunity to remain productive and to maintain a sense of purpose.

If you're sick now, you may be disabled, but if you haven't started ART yet your disability should be temporary—you'll get a lot better once you start treatment. HIV infection can sometimes lead to permanent disability despite treatment, especially in people with advanced disease or in those who develop severe complications that have long-lasting consequences. If you feel you can't work, talk to your provider, a social worker, or a case manager. You may qualify for temporary or permanent disability payments either through your employer, private disability insurance, **Social Security Disability Insurance (SSDI)**, or **Supplemental Security Income (SSI)**. If you intend to keep working but expect frequent absences due to illness or medical visits or health problems, consider filing for benefits under the **Family Medical Leave Act (FMLA)**, which will protect your job during those absences. Information on FMLA is available online or through your employer's human resources department.

Many HIV-positive people are now doing well but continue to receive permanent disability payments because of complications that happened years ago. Some of them aren't working, while others have chosen to give up their disability and go back to work. This can be a tough decision. It's hard to go back to work after years of not working, to explain long gaps in your employment history to a prospective employer, to give up a steady income, and to give up other benefits that often come with being on disability, including Medicaid. On the other hand, disability isn't guaranteed for life. Applications have to be renewed frequently, and unless your medical records indicate that you're *currently* disabled, the checks could stop. (For example, if the note from your last doctor visit says, "Doing great with no medical problems. Just returned from an enjoyable ski trip in the Rockies," good luck justifying your renewal application!)

NOW THAT YOU KNOW

Social Security Disability Insurance (SSDI)

A monthly Social Security benefit for disabled people who have worked in the past and have paid a minimum amount of Social Security taxes.

Supplemental Security Income (SSI)

A federal cash assistance program designed to help the aged, blind, and disabled who have little or no income to pay for basic necessities.

Family Medical Leave Act (FMLA)

A federal law that allows people to take time off work without fear of termination or loss of benefits to deal with their own serious or chronic medical problems or those of their family members. People who need this protection must file paperwork with their employers in advance.

Routine HIV testing is now recommended for all adults and adolescents, which means that almost everyone should know his or her HIV status.

If you feel you're able to return to work after a period of time on disability, there are federal and state transition programs that offer return-to-work programs and benefits. If you're wrestling with this decision, talk it over with your provider, social worker, or case manager.

Mike's comment:

When I was diagnosed, I was sick enough to get SSDI benefits. SSDI stinks. The pay is bad, for one thing. And wait until you meet a prospective partner who asks, "So, what do you do?" Medicare doesn't kick in until you've been getting SSDI for 2 years, so I didn't have insurance, which was worrisome. When my health improved, I returned to work, and I'm glad I did. Work gives me a sense of purpose. It's fun, and the pay is better. When Mr. Right asked me where I work, I didn't have to look down at my shoes and mumble.

Rose's comment:

Working makes me feel like I'm making a contribution. I'm a part of society and am living a normal life. Not everyone can work, but, for me, it's part of my therapy and keeps me alive. My work gives me a goal and a purpose. It's also fun to prove people wrong who told me I'd be too sick to work.

Fourth-generation HIV tests

HIV tests that measure both antigen and antibody, allowing them to detect HIV infection sooner after infection than older antibody tests

Sexually transmitted infections (STIs)

Infections transmitted from person to person through sexual activity. Also called sexually transmitted diseases (STDs).

Hepatitis B

An acute or chronic viral infection of the liver caused by the hepatitis B virus (HBV).

6. But I *don't* know! Should I get tested?

If you're reading this book and asking this question, the answer is *yes*! Routine HIV testing is recommended for *all* adults and adolescents, which means that *everyone* should know his or her HIV status. You could disregard this recommendation if you've never had sex or shared needles, but in general we'd be a lot better off if we stopped worrying about "risk factors" and just tested everybody. We have a simple, cheap, highly accurate test for a disease that's spread from person to person, is highly treatable, and is fatal if untreated. It's tragic that about 1 in 5 HIV-positive Americans don't know they're infected, leading to unnecessary death, illness, and transmission to others.

People often get tested because they're afraid they might have been infected from a specific event, and they often obsess about the "window period": the time between infection and a positive test results. With the older HIV tests, most people had positive result within 2–8 weeks, and between 97% and 99.7% were positive within 3 months. The newer tests (**fourth-generation HIV tests**), which measure both HIV antigen *and* antibody, detect HIV earlier. Ninety-five percent of recently infected people will have positive results within 1–8 weeks (Question 15).

If you're sexually active—and especially if you're having unprotected sex—it makes more sense to get tested routinely every 6 to 12 months rather than try to time the test based on the exposure, which can drive you—and your medical provider—crazy.

Having just recommended that *everyone* get tested, it seems redundant to list other reasons for testing, but here goes. Testing is *especially* recommended for people who've had a **sexually transmitted infection** (**STI**), **hepatitis B, hepatitis C, tuberculosis** (**TB**), **shingles** (**herpes zoster**), or problems that could be caused by HIV infection, such as weight loss or chronic diarrhea. HIV testing should be performed in anyone with lymphoma or unexplained **thrombocytopenia** (low platelet count), anemia (low red blood cell count), or **leukopenia** (low white blood cell count). All pregnant women should be tested, because treatment can prevent transmission to their infants.

Hepatitis C

An acute or chronic viral infection of the liver caused by the hepatitis C virus (HCV).

Tuberculosis (TB)

A bacterial disease caused by *Mycobacterium tuberculosis*. TB most often causes lung disease but can affect any part of the body.

Shingles (herpes zoster)

A painful, blistering rash, usually occurring in a linear band on one side of the body, caused by reactivation of the chickenpox virus (varicella zoster virus, VZV).

Thrombocytopenia

A disorder in which there is an abnormally low number of platelets in the blood.

Leukopenia

A decrease in the number of white blood cells found in blood.

NOW THAT YOU KNOW

PART TWO

The Basics

What's the difference between HIV and AIDS?

How is HIV spread?

How can HIV infection be prevented?

More...

7. What is HIV?

HIV stands for "**h**uman **i**mmunodeficiency **v**irus," the virus that causes **AIDS** (**a**cquired **i**mmunodeficiency **s**yndrome). The difference between HIV infection and AIDS is discussed in Question 10. HIV is passed from person to person through sexual contact, blood exposure, childbirth, and breastfeeding (Question 12).

It's time to take a brief detour into the basic science of the **life cycle** of HIV—I promise to make it short. For even more details, see Question 29, and refer to **Figure 1** because a picture will make this easier to understand.

HIV

Human immunodeficiency virus, the virus that causes HIV infection and AIDS.

AIDS

Acquired immunodeficiency syndrome, a more advanced stage of HIV infection, defined by having a CD4 count below 200 or one of a list of AIDS indicator conditions (see Table 1).

Life cycle

In HIV infection, the stages that the virus goes through, starting with its entry into human cells and ending with the release of new virus particles into the blood.

Retrovirus

A virus that contains RNA and that can turn RNA into DNA through reverse transcription using viral enzymes. HIV is a retrovirus.

Enzymes

Proteins that carry out a biological function. Examples of enzymes carried by HIV include reverse transcriptase, integrase, and protease. Each plays a role in allowing the virus to reproduce, and each is a target for antiretroviral therapy.

Figure 1
The HIV Life Cycle

HIV is a **retrovirus**, a virus that contains **enzymes** (proteins) that can turn **RNA**, its genetic material, into DNA. It's called a retrovirus because this is the reverse of the normal process, in which DNA is converted through the process of **transcription** into RNA. After infection, HIV RNA gets turned into DNA by the **reverse transcriptase** (RT) enzyme, an enzyme that comes with the virus. That viral DNA is then inserted into the DNA of human cells. The viral DNA can then be translated into viral proteins, which form new viruses that go on to infect new cells. Unfortunately, it can also remain latent in long-lived cells (**reservoirs**) such

RNA

Ribonucleic acid, the genetic material of the HIV virus. Viral RNA gets turned into DNA by reverse transcriptase, and the viral DNA then gets inserted into the DNA of human cells. DNA is later transcribed back into RNA, which in turn gets translated into the proteins that are used to make new virus particles.

Transcription

The process of turning DNA into RNA.

Reverse transcriptase (RT)

An enzyme contained within the HIV virus that can turn viral RNA into DNA so it can be inserted into the DNA of human cells. A reverse transcriptase inhibitor blocks this process.

Reservoir

A cell that can harbor viral DNA for long periods of time, maintaining latent infection.

THE BASICS

The HIV Life Cycle

1. **Entry**: CD4 attachment, coreceptor finding, and fusion. HIV begins its life cycle when it attaches to a CD4 receptor and then binds to one of two co-receptors (CR5 or CXCR4) on the surface of the CD4 cell. The envelope (coating) of the virus then fuses with the CD4 cell. After fusion, the virus inserts its RNA (genetic material) into the host cell.

2. **Reverse Transcription**: An HIV enzyme (protein) called reverse transcriptase converts the RNA of the virus into HIV DNA.

3. **Integration**: The newly formed HIV DNA enters the nucleus of the CD4 cell, where an HIV enzyme called integrase inserts it into the human DNA of the CD4 cell. The DNA of the virus can remain hidden for many years in resting CD4 cells, or can be used to create new virus in activated CD4 cells.

4. **Transcription and translation**: In an activated CD4 cell, the HIV DNA is transcribed into RNA, which is then translated into HIV proteins.

5. **Assembly**: An HIV enzyme called protease cuts long chains of HIV proteins into smaller individual proteins. New virus particles are assembled from the smaller HIV proteins and copies of HIV RNA.

6. **Budding**: The newly assembled virus buds push out from the CD4 cell. The new copies of HIV are now free to infect other cells.

Adapted with permission from AIDSinfo, a DHHS information service managed by NIH.

Resting CD4 cells

CD4 cells that live a long time and can harbor HIV DNA, which can't be affected by ART because the cell is not replicating, and thus are an important reservoir of latent HIV.

Pandemic

A global epidemic.

Epidemic

The appearance of new cases of disease (especially an infectious disease) in a human population at a higher rate than would be expected.

Vaccine (vaccination)

A substance that is given, usually by injection, but sometimes by mouth or by nasal spray, to stimulate the immune system to make antibodies against a bacterial or viral pathogen.

HIV-1

The most common form of HIV worldwide.

as **resting CD4 cells** or brain cells, where it can't be reached by antiretroviral drugs. HIV's ability to remain latent is what allows it to persist for life, even with effective treatment. It's what has kept us from finding a cure so far (Question 14).

When it's not treated, HIV infection causes progressive damage to the immune system and is almost universally fatal. It is the world's most serious **pandemic** (a global **epidemic**), and there are no immediate prospects for either a cure or a preventive **vaccine**. Fortunately, treatment today is highly effective, and deaths from HIV disease are now mostly preventable in countries where therapy is available and affordable.

8. Where did HIV come from?

Research now shows that **HIV-1***, the most common type of HIV worldwide, first infected humans in sub-Saharan Africa at some point in the first half of the 20th century. It was transmitted from chimpanzees when people came into contact with their blood through hunting or butchering. HIV probably remained confined to Africa for many decades, in part because travel within and from Africa was uncommon then. We have definite proof of human HIV infection in Africa dating back to 1959.

The virus eventually spread beyond Africa, probably entering the United States in the mid- to late-1970s. Unusual cases of rare infections and cancers began to be seen in gay and bisexual men between 1979 and 1981, and the AIDS epidemic is said to have begun when these reports first appeared in medical journals in 1981,

---

*HIV-2 is a related but less common virus found almost exclusively in West Africa. Standard blood tests will detect both viruses.

making it clear that there was an emerging epidemic. The HIV virus was discovered in 1983, leading to a blood test and eventually to treatment.

The disease was originally reported in gay and bisexual men, but the "risk groups" were later expanded to include injection drug users, hemophiliacs, and Haitians. It eventually became clear that "risk behaviors" were more important than "risk groups." People could be infected through unprotected sex, exposure to infected blood, or through childbirth or breastfeeding. It's estimated that more than 35 million children and adults were infected with HIV worldwide as of 2013.

9. How does HIV make you sick?

HIV causes illness mainly by damaging the immune system. It can infect many human cells, but the most important target is the **CD4 cell** (also known as the **CD4 lymphocyte** or **T-helper cell**). The CD4 cell is a type of **white blood cell** (**WBC**) that is responsible for controlling or preventing infection with many common viruses, bacteria, fungi, and parasites, as well as some cancers. HIV infection leads to destruction of CD4 cells. Over time, the number of CD4 cells (the CD4 count) declines. Although it may take years, the CD4 count eventually becomes so low that there aren't enough cells to fight certain infections or cancers, which allows complications to occur. The speed at which the CD4 count falls varies from person to person and depends on a number of factors, including genetic characteristics, characteristics of the viral strain, and the amount of virus in the blood (viral load).

CD4 cell (CD4 lymphocyte, or T-helper cell)

A type of lymphocyte (a type of whit blood cell) that can be infected by HIV. CD4 cells fight certain infections and cancers. The number of CD4 cells (CD count) declines wit untreated HIV infection, which leads to immunosuppressio

White blood cell (WBC)

A type of blood cell that helps fight infection. CD4 cells are a type of lymph cyte, which is a typ of white blood cell.

Immune activation

A general stimulation of the immune system that can be caused by a variety of infections, including HIV infection. In the case of HIV, it is thought to cause the decline in CD4 count that occurs with time.

The reason for the loss of CD4 cells still isn't completely understood. It's not simply a matter of HIV infecting and directly killing the cells, because the proportion of cells that are actually infected is small. We now know that HIV infection causes a chronic **immune activation** (stimulation of the immune system), which may be responsible for the reduction in the number of CD4 cells. Chronic inflammation may also increase the long-term risk of certain medical conditions, such as coronary heart disease, cancers, or other conditions that become more common as we age (Questions 47 and 61).

In addition to damaging the immune system, HIV can directly affect many of the body's organs, such as the nervous system (Question 73) and the kidneys (Question 49). It can also cause weight loss, night sweats, and diarrhea (Question 11). When deaths due to AIDS were common, it was often said that people didn't die of HIV itself, but of one of its complications, such as a cancer or infection. While that was technically true in most cases, HIV infection was still the underlying problem that led to death from AIDS.

Immunodeficiency (or immuno-suppression)

A state in which the immune system is damaged or impaired, either from birth (congenital immunodeficiency) or acquired, as in HIV infection.

Syndrome

A collection of signs or symptoms that frequently occur together but that may or may not be caused by a single disease.

10. What's the difference between HIV and AIDS?

Everyone who has AIDS has HIV infection, but not everyone with HIV infection has AIDS. AIDS stands for acquired immunodeficiency syndrome. It's "acquired" because you only get it by being infected with HIV from someone else who has it. "**Immunodeficiency**" means it causes damage to the immune system. It's a "**syndrome**" because in the years before HIV was discovered and identified as the cause of AIDS, we recognized a collection of symptoms and complications, including infections and cancers that occurred in people who had common risk factors.

The term *AIDS* was coined in 1982. HIV hadn't been discovered yet, so there was no way to know whether people were infected until they were sick. Someone was said to have AIDS if he (and it was mostly men in those days) developed one of a long list of **opportunistic infections** (**OIs**) and cancers that don't occur in people with healthy immune systems (Question 53). After HIV was discovered and a test became available, the definition of AIDS changed so that having a positive HIV test was required. In 1993, the **Centers for Disease Control and Prevention** (**CDC**) expanded the definition of AIDS to include people with CD4 counts of less than 200. The current **AIDS case definition** is shown in **Table 1**.

Avoid the term "full-blown AIDS." It's old fashioned, unnecessarily scary, and doesn't mean anything other than AIDS. In fact, the term AIDS isn't useful either. If you're HIV-positive, the disease you have is **HIV infection** (or **HIV disease**). AIDS just refers to a more advanced stage of that disease. Treatment can prevent HIV infection from turning into AIDS, and it can restore the health of people with AIDS. In the eyes of the people who keep track of the epidemic, once you have AIDS, you'll always have AIDS. But what should matter to you and your provider is how you're doing *now*.

Opportunistic infection (OI)

An infection that takes advantage of immunodeficiency.

Centers for Disease Control and Prevention (CDC)

A branch of the federal government, within the U.S. Department of Health and Human Services (HHS), that is charged with tracking, preventing, and controlling health problems in the United States, including infectious diseases such as HIV.

AIDS case definition

The criteria used by the CDC to classify someone as having AIDS.

HIV infection (or HIV disease)

The name for the disease caused by HIV infection. AIDS is a late stage of HIV infection.

Table 1 AIDS Indicator Conditions (CDC AIDS Case Definition, 1993)

Candidal esophagitis [65]* (or candidiasis of the respiratory tract, which is rare)

Cervical cancer, invasive [61, 81]

Coccidioidomycosis involving an organ other than the lungs [57]

Cryptococcosis involving an organ other than the lungs [57]

Cryptosporidiosis with diarrhea for at least 1 month [66, 90]

CMV disease involving an organ other than the liver, spleen, or lymph nodes [58]

Herpes simplex with ulcers lasting more than 1 month [89] or with
   esophagitis [65] or infection of the respiratory tract (rare)

Histoplasmosis involving an organ other than the lungs [57]

HIV-associated dementia [73]

Isosporiasis (a parasitic disease that is uncommon in the United States) with diarrhea for at least 1 month [66]

Kaposi's sarcoma [61]

Lymphoma [61]

Mycobacterium avium complex (MAC) [55], *Mycobacterium kansasii,* or other
   mycobacterial infection involving organs other than the lungs

Tuberculosis [59]

Pneumocystis pneumonia (PCP) [54]

Pneumonia, bacterial: two or more episodes in 1 year [67]

Progressive multifocal leukoencephalopathy (PML) [73]

Salmonella with bloodstream infection, recurrent [66]

Toxoplasmosis [56]

Wasting syndrome (greater than 10% weight loss plus chronic diarrhea,
   weakness, or fever lasting more than 30 days) [69]

* Numbers in brackets refer to questions in which the topics are discussed.
Source: Reproduced from the Centers for Disease Control and Prevention.

11. What are the stages of HIV infection?

The first stage of HIV infection, occurring a few weeks after transmission, is called **primary HIV infection** or **acute retroviral syndrome** (**ARS**) (Question 16). During ARS, standard HIV tests, especially antibody tests, are often negative, but the amount of virus in the blood (measured by the viral load) is extremely high, making it easy to transmit HIV to others.

ARS resolves on its own and is followed by a latent stage, usually called **asymptomatic HIV infection**. People generally feel fine during that stage, although their **lymph nodes** may be enlarged (**lymphadenopathy**), and some common conditions can occur more often or be more severe, including vaginal yeast infections, herpes, or shingles.

Some people develop symptoms of HIV infection before actually developing AIDS. This stage is referred to as **symptomatic HIV infection** (formerly **AIDS-related complex**, or **ARC**). Symptoms include weight loss, oral **thrush** (a **yeast** infection in the mouth), persistent diarrhea, night sweats, and fatigue.

You have AIDS if your CD4 count falls below 200 (whether or not you have symptoms) or when an **AIDS-indicator condition** (or **AIDS-defining condition**) has been diagnosed (see Table 1). Most people reach a CD4 count of 200 before developing complications, so a low CD4 count is the most common reason for an AIDS diagnosis. As the CD4 count declines further, the list of possible complications grows. We sometimes refer to someone with a CD4 count below 50 as having **advanced HIV infection**.

THE BASICS

Primary HIV infection

The stage of HIV infection that occurs shortly after infection.

Acute retroviral syndrome (ARS)

A collection of symptoms, such as fever, rash, and swollen lymph nodes, that most people experience during primary infection, shortly after they're infected.

Asymptomatic HIV infection

An early stage of HIV infection in which infected people have a positive test but no symptoms.

Lymph nodes

Structures of the human body that are part of the immune system, acting as filters that collect and destroy bacteria and viruses.

Lymphadenopathy

Swollen or enlarged lymph nodes ("glands").

Symptomatic HIV infection

A stage of HIV infection in which people have symptoms caused by HIV, such as weight loss, diarrhea, or thrush, but have not yet developed an AIDS indicator condition.

AIDS-related complex (ARC)

An old term, no longer used, for the stage of HIV disease in which people have symptoms but have not yet developed AIDS. Now referred to as "symptomatic HIV infection."

Thrush

Oral candidiasis, a yeast infection involving the mouth, presenting with white/yellow curd-like plaques on the palate, gums, or the back of the throat.

Yeast

A group of microorganisms that can sometimes cause human infections, ranging from minor (oral thrush, vaginitis) to severe (cryptococcal meningitis). All yeasts are fungi.

If it's not diagnosed and treated, HIV infection almost always progresses from early stages to late stages, eventually resulting in death. Treatment can move you from a late stage back to an early stage. Having AIDS or advanced HIV infection is not a good thing, but HIV infection is treatable at *any* stage.

12. How is HIV spread?

There are only a few ways in which HIV can be spread:

- *Sexual transmission.* For HIV to be spread through sex, the semen, vaginal fluids, or blood of an infected person must enter the body of an uninfected person. This usually happens through vaginal or anal intercourse. The risk is greatest if the "insertive" partner (the "top") is positive, but the top can be infected by the receptive partner (the "bottom") too. Transmission through oral sex is much less common, but it can happen. (For a more detailed discussion of the risks of specific sexual activities and reducing sexual risk, see Questions 13 and 86.)

- *Blood exposure.* HIV can be transmitted through transfusion, though the risk is virtually nonexistent in places where the blood supply is tested. Far more commonly, it's transmitted through injection drug use, when negative users share needles or syringes ("works") with positive users. Healthcare workers have been infected when they've been stuck with needles containing infected blood or when their eyes, nose, or open cuts have been splashed with blood or body fluids from an HIV-positive patient.

- *Childbirth and breastfeeding.* HIV-infected women can pass HIV to their infants during childbirth (usually at the time of labor or shortly before) or by breastfeeding (see Question 76). Infants aren't infected at the time of conception, so an HIV-positive man can only infect the infant indirectly, by infecting the mother.

HIV isn't spread through contact with saliva, urine, sweat, or feces, and contrary to popular belief, it is *not* transmitted by mosquitoes, exposure of body fluids to intact skin, holding hands, kissing, hugging, sharing drinking glasses or eating utensils, mutual masturbation, or having naughty thoughts!

13. How can HIV infection be prevented?

HIV is a *completely* preventable disease. Here's what you need to know about prevention, organized by the type of transmission:

- *Sexual transmission, HIV-negative people.* It doesn't get any safer than abstinence. But while this approach has its supporters, it's not acceptable to everyone, and even among the most vocal proponents of abstinence, "sex happens." The next best alternatives are to (1) limit the number of sexual partners; (2) engage in sexual activities other than anal or vaginal intercourse; (3) avoid getting semen, pre-seminal fluid ("pre-cum"), and vaginal fluids in your mouth or eyes; (4) use condoms when you *do* have intercourse; (5) use **pre-exposure prophylaxis** (**PrEP**), especially if you're not always using condom. For more details on safer sexual practices, see Question 86. HIV-negative people should play it safe regardless of what they're told about their partners' status. Partners don't always know or reveal their current status, or their status may change.

AIDS indicator condition (or AIDS-defining condition)

One of a list of conditions, including opportunistic infections and malignancies, that is used by the CDC to determine who has AIDS (see Table 1).

Advanced HIV infection

The most advanced stage of HIV infection, usually in people with CD4 counts below 50 or 100.

Pre-exposure prophylaxis (PrEP)

A form of HIV prevention in which antiretroviral medications are taken by HIV-negative individuals to prevent infection.

If you're HIV-negative and you're not always using condoms during sex, PrEP has been shown to be a highly effective way to prevent HIV infection. This currently involves taking Truvada (a pill containing two antiretroviral agents, tenofovir and emtricitabine) once daily to prevent transmission. It won't prevent other sexually transmitted infections, but it will probably keep you from getting HIV, provided you take it regularly. New forms of PrEP are being studied, including long-acting injections. Intermittent or "on-demand" PrEP (taken only around the time of sexual activity) is also being studied, and there were some promising results from a French study. However, the men in that study were taking intermittent PrEP so often that it may not have been much different from continuous PrEP.

Another new approach is the use of vaginal or rectal microbicide (virus-killing) gels, used as sexual lubricants. These are being studied and are at least partially effective, but aren't yet available commercially.

- *Sexual transmission, HIV-positive people.* If you're HIV-positive, it's your responsibility to never infect anyone else (regardless of the behavior or preferences of your partners). Condoms are effective when used regularly and correctly, but they don't work when left unopened in the nightstand drawer. Even more important than condoms is being on effective ART with an undetectable viral load (Questions 28 and 86), which is the most important way for positive people to avoid infecting others.

- *Drug use.* The best way to prevent infection from drug use is to get treatment to help you stop using. But if you're going to use drugs, don't share needles and syringes. That can be easier said than done, especially in places that don't have needle exchange programs. If you do share syringes and needles, decontaminate them with bleach after every use. PrEP has also been shown to protect drug users against HIV infection.

- *Transmission to infants.* All pregnant women should be tested for HIV infection. Treatment during pregnancy is almost 100% effective at preventing transmission to the baby (Question 76). HIV-positive women should not breastfeed their babies.

Don't spend time worrying about obscure ways of getting infected. The simple fact is that if all HIV-positive people were diagnosed and on effective ART, the HIV epidemic would come to an end. Short of that, we can achieve almost the same outcome with broader use of condoms, PrEP, and needle exchange.

14. Why isn't there a cure?

Given how long the disease has been around, it may seem strange that we haven't found a cure for HIV infection yet. Conspiracy theorists argue that a cure exists but is being suppressed by profit-motivated drug companies or by evil governments trying to cull their populations of "less desirable" elements. I'll leave that discussion for later (Question 98), and will talk about science here.

It may surprise you to learn that there is only one viral disease that has ever been cured with medical treatment—hepatitis C (Question 79). All other viral diseases either kill you quickly (Ebola virus), get better on their own (the common cold), remain dormant in your body forever (herpes), or are preventable with vaccination (measles). The fact that HIV hides out by inserting its DNA into long-lived human cells makes it an especially difficult problem to tackle.

It's also worth noting that most of the other diseases that we suffer from in the developed world are *also* chronic, incurable, but treatable diseases. Think of diabetes, coronary artery disease, congestive heart failure, arthritis. None of them is curable, but all of them are manageable ... though they tend to be harder to manage than HIV infection.

Since writing the first edition of this book, I've become more optimistic about the possibility of a cure. You may have heard about Timothy Ray Brown, "the Berlin patient," an HIV-positive man with leukemia who appears to have been cured of HIV after getting a bone marrow transplant using marrow from a donor who was genetically immune to HIV infection because of the **delta 32 deletion**, the absence of CCR5 coreceptors on the surface of the CD4 cell (see Question 27). Of course, this is not the cure we're looking for. Bone marrow transplants are expensive, risky procedures, and people who get them require lifelong immunosuppression to prevent rejection. But Brown's experience tells us that cure is possible and may point us to safer ways to achieve this goal.

There are a number of cure mechanisms that are being studied. **Latency-reversing agents** are drugs that activate or "wake up" infected resting CD4 cells. They're being studied in a "**shock and kill**" approach, where you attack the replicating virus with antiretroviral drugs after activating it with latency-reversing agents. Genetically modifying CD4 cells to make them uninfectable— like the cells that Brown received in his bone marrow

Delta 32 deletion

A genetic condition resulting in the absence of CCR5 coreceptor on the CD4 cell. Individuals who are heterozygous for this deletion (the mutation is present in only one copy of the gene) can be infected by HIV but progress more slowly. Those who are homozygous (the mutation is present in both copies of the gene) cannot be infected by R5 virus, the most common form of circulating HIV.

Latency-reversing agents

Drugs being studied in experimental cure strategies that activate HIV-infected resting CD4 cells in order to eliminate the latent reservoir.

"Shock and kill"

An experimental cure strategy in which HIV-infected resting CD4 cells are first activated by latency-reversing agents, allowing the virus to be treated with antiretroviral therapy.

transplant—could prevent HIV from infecting new cells. Immune-based therapies and therapeutic vaccines could help the immune system fight HIV on its own.

A cure could be "sterilizing" (the virus is completely eradicated) or "functional" (HIV is still present, but the immune system keeps it under control without ART). Cure and eradication research is now a high priority at the National Institutes of Health (NIH) and world-wide. Provided we continue to generously fund scientific research (not always a safe assumption these days), the search for a cure will continue to be the focus of some of our best scientists.

In the meantime, it would be a mistake to look at cure as the only measure of success. In just 15 years, we saw HIV infection go from being an almost universally fatal, untreatable illness to a manageable, chronic disease—and treatment became easier and better in the years that followed. A cure will be a scientific breakthrough of unprecedented proportions; until then, we'll have to be content with triumphant, unparalleled success.

In about 15 years, we saw HIV infection go from being an almost universally fatal, untreatable illness to a manageable, chronic disease.

THE BASICS

PART THREE

Diagnosis

How is HIV infection diagnosed?

How do I know if I've been recently infected?

What if all of my tests are negative but
I'm sure that I'm infected?

More…

15. How is HIV infection diagnosed?

If you already know you're positive, you can skip this section, which was written for readers who don't know their status or have questions about testing.

Tests to diagnose HIV infection are *highly* accurate. The traditional strategy using the older, third-generation antibody tests was to first do an **enzyme-linked immunoassay** (**ELISA** or **EIA**). A negative ELISA usually means you aren't infected, though it could be negative if you'd been infected very recently. If the ELISA is positive, the lab automatically runs a confirmatory test called a **Western blot** (**WB**). If both tests are positive, you're infected. False-positive tests are extremely rare. When they happen, it's usually due to a clerical error: a mislabeled tube or the wrong name on the lab report.

An **indeterminate HIV test** means the ELISA is positive and the WB is not completely negative, but not fully positive, either. This can occur for one of two reasons. First, you might have been recently infected and are in the process of **seroconversion** (development of a positive WB). Second, you might be negative but just happen to have an indeterminate test for reasons that will probably never be determined. If you're seroconverting, the test almost always becomes positive within a month, so if it's still indeterminate 1 to 3 months later and you have an undetectable viral load, you're not infected and you don't need more testing.

Most people develop **antibodies** within 2 to 8 weeks after infection, and virtually 100% are positive within 3 months. We're now moving away from antibody tests in favor of fourth-generation tests, which detect both HIV antibodies and **antigens** (proteins on the surface

---

Enzyme-linked immunoassay (ELISA or EIA)

Traditionally, the initial antibody test used to diagnosed HIV infection. Positive tests were confirmed with Western blot assays.

Western blot (WB)

Traditionally, the confirmatory test used to diagnosed HIV infection in people who tested positive for HIV antibodies by ELISA.

Indeterminate HIV test

This occurs when the EIA is positive but the Western blot contains some bands that are seen with HIV infection, though not enough to make a diagnosis.

Seroconversion

The process of developing an antibody to an infectious agent. In the case of HIV, it occurs shortly after primary infection.

Antibodies

Proteins used by the immune system to fight infection. Antibodies are formed after exposure to antigens—foreign substances such as viruses or bacteria.

of the virus). These tests can detect HIV earlier, short-ening the **window period**; using the new tests, 95% of infected persons will test positive within 1 to 8 weeks of infection.

Viral load testing (HIV RNA) is positive even sooner than antigen-based tests and can be used to diagnose acute infection. It's not a good diagnostic test for HIV in general, because it can be negative (**undetectable**) in people who are infected, and it can give a positive (**detectable** at low levels) result in people who aren't infected. It *is* a useful test to diagnose acute retroviral syndrome in people with symptoms (Question 16).

Rapid tests can give you a result within a few min-utes. A rapid fourth-generation test is available as well. **Home tests** are also available. The *Home Access* test (www.homeaccess.com) uses blood from a finger stick, which is mailed in and results are given over the phone. *OraQuick* (www.oraquick.com) uses an oral swab and provides immediate results. Follow the instructions to the letter, because *OraQuick* has been somewhat less sensitive when performed by lay people than by labora-tory or medical personnel. Positive tests should always be confirmed by a lab-based test.

16. How do I know if I've been recently infected?

Most people feel sick within a few weeks of HIV infec-tion. This is called primary infection or acute retroviral syndrome (ARS) (Question 11). The illness may be mild and brief or it may be severe enough to require hospi-talization. In most cases, the symptoms are similar to those of mononucleosis. They can include fever, muscle

Antigens

Proteins from organisms, such as bacteria or viruses, that stim-ulate an immune response.

Window period

The period between infection and formation of antibodies leading to a positive HIV test (serology).

Undetectable

A term used to describe a viral load that is too low to be mea-sured by a viral load test. An undetectable viral load is below 20 to 400, depending on which test is being used.

Detectable

A word used to describe a viral load that is high enough to be measured by a viral load test. A detectable viral load is one that is above 50 to 400, depend-ing on which test is being used.

Rapid tests

HIV tests that provide an answer within a few minutes, using either blood or saliva. Positive tests must be confirmed with stan-dard serologies.

DIAGNOSIS

Home tests

An HIV blood or oral test that can be performed at home.

Bell's palsy

A paralysis of one side of the face that can be caused by a variety of infections, including acute HIV infection.

Aseptic meningitis

Meningitis that is not caused by a bacterium that can be grown in culture. Can be caused by viruses (including HIV during ARS) or drugs.

Guillain-Barré syndrome

Progressive muscle paralysis starting in the legs and moving upward, sometimes seen during acute retroviral syndrome.

Myopathy

An inflammation of muscles causing muscle pain and weakness, sometimes seen with acute retroviral syndrome, high-dose zidovudine, or statin drugs used to lower cholesterol.

Serologies

Blood tests that measures antibodies or antigens to look for evidence of a disease.

aches, fatigue, sore throat, swollen lymph nodes, or rash. Less often, people can develop neurological symptoms, such as **Bell's palsy** (paralysis of one side of the face), **aseptic meningitis**, **Guillain-Barré syndrome** (paralysis that starts in the legs and moves up the body), or **myopathy** (muscle pain and weakness). Sometimes, people with ARS become seriously immunosuppressed and develop opportunistic infections that normally occur only in people with longstanding HIV disease, but this happens rarely.

During ARS, standard HIV test are usually negative or indeterminate. Fourth-generation antibody/antigen tests (Question 15) are more likely to be positive, and the viral load will be very high (in the hundreds of thousands or even millions). If the HIV **serology** is negative and the viral load is undetectable, HIV is not the cause of the symptoms.

Unfortunately, the diagnosis of ARS is too often missed. The symptoms are nonspecific (common to other viral conditions), and many healthcare providers either don't think about ARS or don't know how to diagnosis it. Even if HIV crosses their mind, they may order only a standard HIV antibody test, which is often negative. It's important to diagnose HIV infection at this stage for several reasons. First, people with ARS have extremely high levels of HIV in their blood, semen, and vaginal fluids, making it easy for them spread HIV to others if they don't know they're infected. Second, it's possible to be infected with drug-resistant HIV (virus that isn't suppressed by one or more drugs; see Question 38). The best time to test for transmitted resistance is during ARS (Question 24). Finally, there may be a benefit to starting treatment during ARS rather than waiting. Starting treatment *very* early may reduce the size of the latent reservoir, and it's thought that such people will be the best candidates for a cure, when a cure becomes available.

17. What if all of my tests are negative, but I'm sure that I'm infected?

I don't want to come down too hard on the "worried well"—people who are convinced they have HIV infection despite overwhelming evidence to the contrary. After all, I'm hoping they'll buy so many copies of this book that we'll have to print more for the folks who really *do* have HIV. But the simple fact is that HIV is *not* hard to diagnose. A negative HIV test after the appropriate window period for that test means you're not infected. You don't need a viral load, a CD4 count, a DNA test, or a viral culture. You don't need to see a specialist. You don't need to think about rare subtypes or whether medications you take are causing false-negative tests results.

What you *may* need is a psychiatrist or a psychotherapist. Irrational obsession with disease can be a sign of depression, obsessive-compulsive disorder, or hypochondriasis. Depression and anxiety can cause many of the symptoms that lead the worried well to think they're infected. People may also obsess about HIV infection because it's easier than dealing with more difficult issues like guilt or anxiety about sexuality or infidelity.

HIV is not *hard to diagnose.*

My advice: Buy this book, read this chapter, then put the book down, stay off the Internet, and start addressing the underlying causes for your irrational obsession with HIV infection.

DIAGNOSIS

PART FOUR

Medical Care

How do I find the right medical care?

What are my provider's responsibilities
and what are mine?

How will I pay for medical care?

More...

18. How do I find the right medical care?

The choice of a medical provider may be the most important one you make, so make it carefully. Treating HIV infection is complex; it's not something that should be attempted by providers without experience and training. Studies have shown that people treated by HIV experts stay healthier and live longer than those managed by nonexperts. Mistakes made by inexperienced clinicians early in the course of therapy can lead to drug resistance that never goes away. I know of doctors who will refer a kid with zits to a dermatologist, but they'll try to manage HIV by themselves. Don't let that happen to you! If your doctor says he hasn't managed many HIV-positive patients, but he went to a dinner talk once and "it can't be that hard," run the other way!

I use the term "expert," because there's technically no such thing as an "HIV specialist." A specialist is someone who has passed a specialty board exam, and there is no such exam for HIV. An HIV expert is a clinician with lots of HIV experience who keeps up with the latest research and developments in the field. Some infectious disease specialists are HIV experts, but some aren't. There are general internists and family practitioners who *are* HIV experts. Experts don't even have to be doctors: There are expert nurse practitioners and physician assistants, which is why I tend to use terms like "clinician" or "healthcare provider" rather than "doctor" in this book.

Finding expert care can be tricky. If you have a primary medical provider, he or she may be able to refer you to someone. Ask a **case manager** or someone at an **AIDS service organization** for a recommendation. Talk

Case manager

A person who helps coordinate your medical care, provides referrals for needed services, and determines whether you qualify for any assistance or entitlement programs.

AIDS service organization (ASO)

An organization that provides services to people with HIV infection.

to infected friends or support group members. Look for an expert in your area on the website for the American Academy of HIV Medicine (www.aahivm.org) or the HIV Medicine Association (www.hivma.org).

Having HIV doesn't mean you have to give up your primary provider. Some HIV experts serve only as consultants to primary providers, while others provide primary medical care themselves. What matters is that your HIV care be directed by an expert, and that the expert and your primary provider communicate with each other.

I've been a big supporter of the Affordable Care Act ("Obamacare"), because it increases the number of Americans with affordable health insurance. However, there can be downsides for people with HIV, who have had access to expert care through the Ryan White Care Act. This program, which provides HIV care to uninsured people, has led to the development of centers across the country that provide outstanding, comprehensive medical care and "wrap-around services" that help people stay in care. With the Affordable Care Act, more HIV-positive patients will become insured and transitioned to Medicaid. They may be forced to receive their care at Federally Qualified Health Centers (FQHCs). There's nothing wrong with FQHCs (I work at one), provided it has clinicians with HIV expertise and some of those same wrap-around services, but not all of them do. In addition, you now have to be careful when you sign up for an insurance plan using the Marketplace, because some plans actively discriminate against HIV-positive people by placing antiretroviral medications on high tiers that require huge copays. Do your homework, preferably with the help of an HIV-savvy case manager or Obamacare "navigator."

People treated by HIV experts stay healthier and live longer than those managed by non-experts.

19. How do I deal with my healthcare provider?

The provider who treats you for HIV infection is going to be an important person in your life for a long time. This is someone you should like, trust, respect, and be able to communicate with. As with any long-term relationship, your first may not be "The One." Don't be afraid to shop around a little. Here are a few questions you should ask when you start a relationship with a new provider:

1. *Are you covered by my insurance plan?* This question is usually answered by the office staff or by someone from your insurance company before you ever see the provider (who may not know).

2. *How much experience do you have with HIV? How do you keep up with the latest advances in the field?* These may seem like awkward questions, but only someone who doesn't have what it takes will answer them defensively.

3. *Will you be my primary provider or will you act as a consultant? Who should I contact about urgent medical problems?* The answer to the questions may be up to you, the provider, or your insurance company, but it's important to clarify them early on.

4. *How often will I see you? When do I get lab work drawn—before the visit or on the same day?* Either is fine, but personally I prefer to have recent lab results available at the time of the appointment, which makes for a more productive visit.

5. *How do I reach you between visits for questions, new problems, or emergencies?* Some providers use email or web portals to communicate with patients; others have special phone-in hours;

others use nurses, physician assistants, or nurse practitioners for first contact. Find out who covers your provider for questions and emergencies when the provider is not on call.

6. *Where would I go if I needed to be hospitalized?* You'd like to think that a great provider would be affiliated with a great hospital, but it doesn't always work that way. Fortunately, hospitalization is no longer inevitable, as it was in the early years of the AIDS epidemic, but it's still worth considering whether you'd be comfortable going to the hospital to which your provider admits patients. Also, it's now common to be cared for by hospitalists when you're an inpatient rather than by your own doctor. Hospitalists are doctors who treat only hospitalized patients, and then turn the care back to the primary care provider after discharge.

20. What are my provider's responsibilities and what are mine?

Because your relationship with your provider should be a partnership, there are mutual responsibilities that both parties should be aware of.

Your Provider's Responsibilities

1. To treat you with respect and to pay attention to your concerns and opinions.

2. To ensure that urgent medical care is available to you at all times.

3. To keep you informed about your health status, your progress, and your prognosis in language you can understand.

4. To tell you about your treatment options and to be willing to provide advice about which option he or she thinks is best.

5. To inform you of important side effects or long-term toxicities of medications and to help you weigh the risks and benefits of therapy (without overwhelming you with a long list of bad things that rarely happen).

Your Responsibilities

1. To treat the provider and staff with respect.

2. To provide a complete history, even if it means tracking down old medical records yourself. Better yet, keep your own records! See **Table 2** for a list of things you should keep track of.

3. To keep appointments or to cancel them with plenty of notice whenever possible.

4. To follow the course of treatment agreed on and to let the provider know about problems early so that treatment can be changed.

5. To be honest about what's going on in your life and with your treatment—even if it means disappointing your provider.

6. To understand that "you can't always get what you want." There is evidence that higher "patient satisfaction" was associated with higher death rates and more medical complications. How to explain this seemingly incomprehensible finding? If I tell my patient that he can't have an antibiotic for his cold, or narcotics for his low back pain, or *Xanax* for his stress, he may be upset and rate me poorly on a satisfaction survey, but I'm practicing good, evidence-based medicine. If I tell an obese smoker that she should lose weight and stop smoking, she may be less

Table 2 Information to Keep Track of and Share with New Providers

Dates

Date of HIV diagnosis

Approximate date of infection, if known (dates of exposure, previous negative tests, acute retroviral syndrome, etc.)

Dates of major complications

Test results (with dates)

CD4 counts

Viral loads

Resistance tests (genotypes and phenotypes)

Hepatitis A, B, and C serologies

Toxoplasma IgG antibody

Syphilis tests

Gonorrhea and chlamydia tests

Pap smears (cervical and/or anal)

Tests for latent TB infection (tuberculin skin test or interferon-gamma releasing assay)

Other tests, if applicable (HLA B*5701, tropism assay, etc.)

Vaccinations (with dates)

Tetanus (dT or Tdap)

Pneumococcal (Pneumovax, Prevnar 13)

Hepatitis A

Hepatitis B

Influenza (flu)

Human papillomavirus vaccine

Travel vaccines

Treatment history

All antiretroviral therapy (with start and stop dates for each drug)

Side effects and allergic reactions

Prophylaxis or treatment for opportunistic infections or complications

Other important information

Emergency contacts

Case manager or social worker

Advance directives (living will, durable power of attorney for health care)

MEDICAL CARE

satisfied than if I tell her everything's fine, but then I wouldn't be practicing good medicine. Your relationship with your provider is a partnership, but it's not exactly an equal one. Your provider is there to give you what you *need* based on evidence and expertise, which may not always be what you *want*.

Mike's comment:

When I showed up at Dr. Gallant's office, I was a lot sicker than I realized. My CD4 count was in the double digits and my viral load was sky-high. I was losing sensation from the waist down. I'd only been infected for about a year and a half and was a fast progressor. What allowed me to live was:

1. *Medicines that work*

2. *A doctor who knows what he's doing (He is the author of this book, after all!)*

3. *Following the treatment plan that I agreed to*

21. How will I pay for medical care?

Because this book is written from a U.S. perspective, the answer is complex. We have never really had a "health-care system" in this country; we've had multiple systems that depend on where you live, how old you are, how much money you make, your immigration status, and whether you're disabled—with lots of people falling through the many large, gaping cracks. Fortunately, having HIV infection has entitled you to benefits that would not be available if you had some other disease.

The Affordable Care Act (ACA, or "Obamacare") has brought us closer to universal coverage, but it still leaves us at the mercy of the insurance companies, some of

HIV care is expensive. The average wholesale price of a year's worth of non-generic ART costs in the range of $28,000 to $35,000 per year, not including medical visits or lab tests. Few people pay for this out of pocket.

which, as I write this, are engaging in discriminatory pricing practices that discourage HIV-positive patients from enrolling in their plans. I've already discussed ways in which the ACA could make it harder for HIV-positive patients to access HIV experts (Question 18).

HIV care is expensive. The average wholesale price of a year's worth of non-generic ART costs in the range of $28,000 to $35,000 per year, not including medical visits or lab tests. Few people pay for this out of pocket. Those with private insurance are generally covered, though some plans require high copays or have limits on medication coverage. There may be government programs or pharmaceutical industry copay assistance programs that can help cover these costs; talk to your case manager or social worker.

If you're uninsured, or if your insurance doesn't cover your medications, you may qualify for the **AIDS Drug Assistance Program (ADAP)** in your state. This is a program that provides HIV medications to people who fall below a specified income level. The coverage provided by ADAP programs varies from state to state. Some states' programs are quite generous, whereas others are skimpier and may have waiting lists or shorter lists of covered medications. Medical visits and lab tests are often paid for by federal **Ryan White Care Act** funds that are received by some HIV providers or treatment centers. As I write this, Ryan White funding remains intact, but its future is uncertain, as I've discussed in Question 18. Finally, the ACA has made it easier for people with HIV infection to qualify for **Medicaid** or private insurance. In some states, Ryan White funds can be used to pay insurance premiums.

MEDICAL CARE

AIDS Drug Assistance Program (ADAP)

A federally funded program that provides antiretroviral medications and other HIV-related medications to those who have no other way to pay for them. The programs are administered by the states, and coverage varies from state to state.

Ryan White Care Act

A government-funded program that provides money on a state or local level to provide care for uninsured people with HIV infection.

Medicaid

An insurance program funded by the federal and state governments that provides coverage for medical care to low-income, uninsured people.

The complexities of insurance, benefits, and entitlements vary too much and change too quickly for me to be able to do them justice in this book. My advice is to talk to an HIV-savvy case manager, social worker, or Obamacare navigator and find out where you stand. You can find them at HIV clinics and AIDS service organizations.

PART FIVE

Getting Started

What does my CD4 count mean?

What is a resistance test, and when should I get one?

What vaccinations do I need?

More...

22. What does my CD4 count mean?

Red blood cell (RBC)

A blood cell that carries oxygen to the organs of the body. If you don't have enough RBCs, you're anemic.

Platelet

A blood cell that helps blood clot. A low platelet count, which can sometimes occur due to HIV infection, can result in easy bleeding or bruising.

Lymphocyte

A type of infection-fighting white blood cell. CD4 cells are a type of lymphocyte.

Prophylaxis

Prevention, usually applied to the use of medications taken to prevent opportunistic infections or to keep them from coming back after they've been treated.

Your blood contains **red blood cells** (**RBCs**), white blood cells (WBCs), and **platelets**. **Lymphocytes** are a type of WBC, and the CD4 cell is a specific type of lymphocyte, the one most affected by HIV. The CD4 count measures the health of your immune system. It should be checked regularly (usually every 3 to 6 months) if you're *not* on therapy because it measures the amount of damage done by HIV and is the most important test for determining the urgency of starting ART (Question 28) and the need for **prophylaxis** (prevention) for opportunistic infections (Question 60). The CD4 count almost always increases with effective ART, but how much it will increase is hard to predict.

Once you're on ART, the viral load is a more important measure of your response to therapy than the CD4 count. If your viral load is undetectable—the goal of therapy—it's unlikely that you would ever make any changes based on the CD4 count. An ideal response to ART is to have an undetectable viral load and a CD4 count above 500. Once you reach that goal, current U.S. guidelines say that continued CD4 count testing is optional, though many patients and providers still think of the viral load and CD4 count as tests that should always be ordered together. In my own practice, I generally order the CD4 count once a year in people who are doing well on ART. I'm not sure why. I guess it's a combination of inertia and patient expectations.

The CD4 count can vary from day to day—even from hour to hour. It can drop temporarily when you're sick or have been vaccinated and can be affected by the way it's processed in the lab. Don't pay too much attention to a single count, and don't get too worried or excited about a single count that's inconsistent with previous counts. It's the *trend* that matters, not one number. When in doubt, you can also look at the **CD4 percent**—the percentage of your lymphocytes that are CD4 cells. This number doesn't vary as much as the CD4 count, so if your CD4 count has changed but your CD4 percent hasn't, chances are it's not an important change. And remember that a high normal CD4 count is no better than a low normal CD4 count. Once it's above 500, it doesn't matter what the number is. Don't be like my patient who freaks out when his CD4 count "falls" from 920 to 880!

CD8 cells (or **CD8 lymphocytes**, or **T-suppressor cells**) are also affected by HIV infection, and we know that having a higher ratio of CD4 cells to CD8 cells (CD4/CD8 ratio) is better than having a lower ratio. But we don't use these numbers to make treatment decisions, because there's nothing you can do with the results other than to take ART. They're not recommended tests; all they do is make CD4 monitoring more expensive.

CD4 percent

The percentage of lymphocytes that are CD4 cells. The CD4 percent is provided whenever a CD4 count is ordered and provides additional information about the state of the immune system.

CD8 cells (or CD8 lymphocytes, or T-suppressor cells)

Another type of lymphocyte affected by HIV infection. Measuring CD8 cells is not necessary, because the CD8 count is not used to make treatment decisions.

23. What's a viral load?

The viral load (viral HIV RNA) measures the amount of HIV in your blood. It's a measure of the activity of the virus and of how well ART is working. It's also used, along with the CD4 count, to help decide the urgency of starting treatment.

The viral load can range from very low (less than 20 copies per milliliter of blood) to very high (millions of copies). It is highest during the acute retroviral syndrome and in people with advanced disease who aren't on treatment. When treatment is effective, the viral load should be undetectable—generally less than 20 in the test that's most commonly used. Having an undetectable viral load doesn't mean there's no virus; it just means that the viral load is too low to be measured by standard blood tests.

Your viral load should be measured about a month after starting or changing therapy, and then routinely—usually every 3 to 4 months. Regular measurements are especially important after starting treatment, because that's how you know whether the drugs are working. If you've been on ART with an undetectable viral load for years, checking it every 6 months is sufficient. The viral load should drop at least ten-fold [1 **log (logarithm)**] during the first month of therapy (e.g., from 100,000 to 10,000), and it should be undetectable within 3 to 6 months, depending on how high it was before you started. The viral load will decline faster if you're taking an integrase inhibitor (Question 29), usually becoming undetectable within 1 to 2 months.

If your viral load is detectable once in a while, don't panic. It may just be a "**blip**"—a single viral load that's detectable at low levels (usually well below 1,000). Blips can result from normal lab variation (no lab test is 100% accurate), so they're generally nothing to be alarmed about, provided you're taking your medications faithfully. We define treatment failure as a viral load that is repeatedly above 200. Of course, you can't be sure it's a blip until you repeat the test, which is important to do, because a detectable viral load can also be a sign of early treatment **failure**.

Log (logarithm)

Another way of expressing viral load results. A viral load of 100,000 is a viral load of five logs; 10,000 is four logs; 1,000 is three logs. A tenfold change in viral load is a one-log change. For example, a drop in viral load from 100,000 to 1,000 is a "two-log drop."

Blip

A single detectable viral load with undetectable viral loads before and after.

Failure

Loss of activity of ART. Includes virologic failure (detectable viral load on therapy), immunologic failure (falling CD4 count on therapy), and clinical failure (worsening symptoms on therapy).

24. What is a resistance test, and when should I get one?

Resistance tests tell you which drugs will work to treat your particular virus. Not all viruses respond to all medications. Resistance tests help your provider choose the best drugs to treat you with. Unlike CD4 counts and viral loads, resistance tests aren't ordered on a regular basis. They're ordered for only two reasons: to find out whether you were infected with resistant virus and to find out whether you've developed **resistance** if your treatment is failing.

You should be tested for resistance as soon as you're diagnosed with HIV, even if you're not starting ART right away. The test is less accurate if it's delayed. Your provider should also order a resistance test if you're failing therapy, to determine which drugs are no longer working and which drugs to use next.

There are two types of resistance tests: **genotype tests** and **phenotype tests**. Genotype tests look for **mutations** (changes) in the genes of the virus that cause resistance to specific drugs. Phenotype tests measure the virus's ability to replicate (multiply or reproduce) in the presence of drugs. Genotype tests are faster and cheaper, but they can be hard to interpret if there are a lot of mutations. Phenotype tests take longer and cost more, but they measure resistance more directly and are better at determining whether a drug still has partial activity despite mutations. We tend to use genotype tests when we expect the results to be fairly straightforward, reserving phenotype tests for people with more extensive resistance.

GETTING STARTED

Resistance

The ability of the virus to replicate despite the presence of antiretroviral medications.

Genotype test

In HIV, a type of resistance test that looks for specific resistance mutations known to cause resistance to antiretroviral drugs.

Phenotype test

A type of resistance test that measures the ability of the virus to replicate in varying concentrations of antiretroviral drugs.

Mutations

Changes in the normal genetic make-up of an organism due to a mistake that occurs during reproduction. In the case of HIV, some mutations can cause resistance, allowing the virus to replicate in the presence of antiretroviral drugs.

Resistance tests tell you which drugs will work to treat your particular virus.

Complete blood count (CBC)

A standard blood test that measures the red and white blood cell counts, hematocrit, hemoglobin, and platelet count.

Hemoglobin

The oxygen-carrying component of red blood cells. Also used as a measure of the amount of red blood cells in the blood.

Hematocrit

A measure of the amount of red blood cells in the blood.

Comprehensive chemistry panel

A standard blood test that measures kidney function, looks for evidence of liver disease, assesses nutritional status, and looks for electrolyte (sodium, potassium) abnormalities.

Hepatitis

Inflammation or infection of the liver.

Resistance tests aren't perfect. The lab may not be able to do the test if your viral load is below 500 to 1,000, and the tests are better at finding out which drugs *won't* work than which ones *will*. Bad news (evidence of resistance) is always believable, but you have to take good news (evidence of sensitivity to drugs) with a grain of salt. They can't always give you reliable information about drugs you've taken in the past, because resistant virus may be present in reservoirs but no longer detectable. Don't ignore old resistance test results. If resistance was detected 5 years ago, it's still there—even if it doesn't show up on a test today.

There are two new types of resistance tests to be aware of. Integrase genotype and phenotype tests look for resistance to drugs classified as integrase inhibitors (see Question 29). They should be ordered in people who are failing therapy with an integrase inhibitor, but are not included in some of the standard resistance tests and must be ordered separately unless you're using a combined assay. The *GenoSure Archive* is a new genotype test that looks for archived resistance: resistance you developed in the past that wouldn't necessarily be detected by standard resistance tests. Unlike other genotype tests, the *GenoSure Archive* doesn't require a minimum viral load. Although we have little clinical experience with it so far, it has the potential to help guide the choice of therapy in people who don't have access to old medical records and resistance tests.

25. What other tests do I need?

Here's a list of important tests. Some are ordered just once, when you're first diagnosed, while others are ordered on a regular basis:

- *Complete blood count (CBC)*. At baseline and every 3 to 6 months to look for anemia (**hemoglobin** and **hematocrit**), low white blood cell count, or platelet problems.

- *Comprehensive chemistry panel*. At baseline and every 3 to 6 months, mainly to assess the liver and kidneys.

- *Hepatitis tests*. Baseline testing for hepatitis A, B, and C and follow-up antibodies for A and B after vaccination to see if it worked (Questions 79 and 80). If the initial tests show evidence of either chronic hepatitis B or C, then you need further testing, including hepatitis B or C viral load tests (**HBV DNA** or **HCV RNA**). In injection drug users or gay men at high risk, HCV testing should be ordered on a regular basis.

- *Tests for sexually transmitted infection*. Tests for syphilis, gonorrhea, and chlamydia at least once a year if you've been sexually active (Question 89).

- *Tuberculosis testing*. **Tuberculin skin test (TST)**, **purified protein derivative (PPD)**, or **interferon-gamma releasing assay (IGRA)** such as *QuantiFERON-TB Gold* to find out whether you've been exposed to the bacterium that causes tuberculosis (Question 59).

- *Toxoplasma IgG antibody*. To find out whether you've been exposed to the parasite that causes **toxoplasmosis** (Question 56).

- *Pap smear*. In women, to look for **cervical dysplasia** (changes in the cells of the

GETTING STARTED

HBV DNA

The "viral load" for hepatitis B, used to make the diagnosis in some people with negative HBV antibodies and to monitor response to hepatitis B therapy.

HCV RNA

The "viral load" for hepatitis C, used to confirm the diagnosis in people with a positive HCV antibody, to make the diagnosis in some people with a negative antibody, and to monitor response to hepatitis C therapy.

Tuberculin skin test (TST or purified protein derivative [PPD])

A skin test used to look for evidence of past exposure to Mycobacterium tuberculosis, the bacterium that causes tuberculosis.

Interferon-gamma releasing assay (IGRA)

A blood test used to detect latent infection with the TB bacterium as an alternative to a tuberculin skin test.

QuantiFERON-TB Gold

The most commonly used IGRA.

Toxoplasmosis

Disease caused by the parasite, *Toxoplasma gondii.*

Anal Pap smear

A diagnostic test to screen for anal dysplasia. Also called "anal cytology.

Pap smear

A diagnostic test used to look for cervical dysplasia and cervical cancer.

Cervical dysplasia

Abnormal cells of the cervix, the mouth of the uterus, caused by human papillomavirus (HPV). If left untreated, it can progress to cervical cancer.

Fasting glucose

Measures blood glucose levels after hours without food.

Lipid panel

A blood test that measures lipid levels in your blood (cholesterol and fats).

Urinalysis

A standard lab test that looks for evidence of protein, sugar, blood, and infection in the urine.

cervix) or cancer. Pap smears should be repeated at least yearly. **Anal Pap smears** should be considered in both women and men, especially those who've had receptive anal sex (Question 81).

- *Fasting glucose and lipid panel*. Before starting ART and periodically after that, especially if you're on HIV drugs that increase cholesterol, triglycerides, and blood sugar (Question 43).

- *Urinalysis*. To look for kidney problems or signs of infection (Question 49). This test should be ordered every 6 months if you're taking a drug regimen that includes tenofovir (*Viread, Truvada, Complera, Atripla,* or *Stribild*).

Other tests that are sometimes ordered include antibodies against CMV (anti-CMV IgG), a chest x-ray, and an HLA B*5701 assay, to find out whether it's safe to take abacavir (see Question 45).

26. What vaccinations do I need?

- **Tetanus toxoid** (**dT** or **Tdap**). Everyone needs a tetanus booster every 10 years. If you haven't had the Tdap, which includes diphtheria and pertussis (whopping cough) vaccines, you need that once, and it's not necessary to wait until you're due for your next tetanus booster.

- **Pneumococcal vaccine**. These vaccines help protect you against **pneumococcus,** a bacterium that causes pneumonia. Start with *Prevnar 13*, followed at least 8 weeks later with two *Pneumovax* doses given 5 years apart. If you received the *Pneumovax* first, wait at least a year before receiving *Prevnar 13*.

- *Hepatitis A vaccine.* If you've never had **hepatitis A** and you're not immune to it (with a positive total or IgG **HAV antibody**), consider getting the two-shot vaccine series with follow-up antibody testing to be sure the vaccine worked. Hepatitis A vaccine is especially important for gay and bisexual men, travelers to resource-limited countries, and people who also have chronic hepatitis B or C.

- *Hepatitis B vaccine.* If you've never had hepatitis B and you're not immune to it (with a positive surface antibody [HBsAb]), you should get the three-part vaccine series with follow-up antibody testing to be sure the vaccine worked. There's also a three-dose combination vaccine (*Twinrix*) that protects you against both hepatitis A and B.

- *Influenza ("flu") vaccine.* A flu shot* is recommended in the fall, not because HIV-positive people get more flu or worse flu than anyone else, but because it's a drag to get the flu. Get the injectable vaccine, not the live-virus nasal spray.

- *Varicella zoster virus (chickenpox) vaccine.* If your CD4 count is above 200, you don't remember having ever had chickenpox or shingles, and you have a negative anti-varicella IgG antibody, consider getting this vaccine.

- *Shingles (herpes zoster) vaccine.* This vaccine is approved for people over 50 and recommended for the general population over 60 by the CDC. It hasn't been approved for HIV-positive people, but we consider it safe if you have a CD4 count above 200.

---

*Not only does the flu vaccine not cause autism, but it also doesn't cause the flu. It's typically given during cold season, so it's inevitable that some people will catch a cold shortly after getting vaccinated and will blame the vaccine. Don't be one of those people!

Tetanus toxoid (dT or Tdap)

Tetanus immunization should be received every 10 years for adults, regardless of HIV status. Tdap (a combination tetanus, diphtheria, pertussis vaccine) should be given once.

Pneumococcal vaccine

A vaccine (Prevnar 13, Pneumovax) recommended for HIV-positive adults to prevent pneumonia caused by pneumococcus.

Pneumococcus

The common name for *Streptococcus pneumoniae*, a frequent cause of bacterial pneumonia.

Hepatitis A

A viral infection of the liver caused by hepatitis A virus (HAV).

HAV antibody

A blood test for hepatitis A. The IgM antibody looks for acute hepatitis; the IgG or total antibody looks for immunity.

Influenza ("flu")

A viral infection caused by influenza virus that causes fever, muscle aches, respiratory symptoms, and gastrointestinal symptoms.

Varicella zoster virus (chickenpox)

The virus that causes chickenpox and shingles (herpes zoster).

Human papillomavirus (HPV)

A sexually transmitted virus that causes abnormal cells (dysplasia) in the cervix, anus, and mouth, which can lead to cancer if not treated.

- *Human papillomavirus (HPV) vaccine.* The best time to get this vaccine is before you've ever had sex, but it's currently recommended for men and women up to the age of 26. It prevents cancers caused by HPV, including cervical and anal cancer (Question 81). Even if you already have HPV-related conditions (anogenital warts, cervical or anal dysplasia), it may still protect you against strains you've haven't been infected with. If you're over 26, you can still consider getting vaccinated, but it's less likely to be covered by your insurance.

Vaccines for international travel are discussed in Question 93.

Vaccines work best when the immune system is strong. If you'll soon be starting ART, the vaccines will be more effective if you wait until after your CD4 count has risen and your viral load is undetectable.

PART SIX

Starting Treatment

How does antiretroviral therapy work?

How do my provider and I choose my first regimen?

Why is adherence so important?

More...

27. How does antiretroviral therapy work?

Antiretroviral drugs don't kill HIV; they stop it from replicating (reproducing itself). If you stop replication, you stop the virus from infecting new cells. Suppressing replication also reduces the immune activation and inflammation that are thought to cause much of the damage to the immune system (Question 9). Turning off replication, immune activation, and inflammation allows the immune system to recover and the CD4 count to increase.

Combination therapy has been a guiding principle since the mid-1990s. The reason for combining several drugs into a single **regimen** or "cocktail" is to prevent resistance. When the virus reproduces, it doesn't do so carefully. It's in a hurry and makes lots of mistakes, which are called mutations. Billions of **virions** (virus particles) are produced each day if you're not on therapy. Because of the high error rate, almost every mutation that *could* occur *does* occur, on a daily basis. Before the days of ART that could fully suppress replication, treatment for HIV involved one or two relatively weak drugs. Mutations that allowed the virus to replicate in the presence of those drugs could appear spontaneously. Those resistant mutants then had an advantage over the original **wild-type virus** (drug-sensitive virus without mutations). Over time, they became selected as the predominant **strain**, and the drugs were no longer effective.

It's far more difficult for the virus to spontaneously develop enough mutations to cause resistance to multiple drugs. When you're taking an ART regimen that includes several active drugs, resistance can only occur when drug levels aren't high enough to keep the virus from replicating, such as when you miss doses.

Antiretroviral drugs don't kill HIV; they stop it from replicating (reproducing itself).

Combination therapy

The use of more than one antiretroviral drug to suppress HIV infection.

Regimen

A combination of antiretroviral drugs.

Virions

Single virus particles.

Wild-type virus

The strain of HIV that occurs "in the wild"—without the presence of antiretroviral drugs that could select for mutations. Generally a non-mutant, drug-sensitive virus.

Strain

In the case of HIV, a type of virus, as in "drug-resistant strain."

While most current ART regimens consist of at least three drugs, there's nothing magic about the number three. It's possible to use fewer drugs if they're potent and if they have a high "resistance barrier," meaning that the virus needs multiple mutations to develop resistance.

28. Should I start treatment?

The short answer is *yes!* The more nuanced answer depends in part on your CD4 count and viral load and whether you're ready to make the kind of commitment that ART requires. Current U.S. guidelines recommend treatment for *everyone* with HIV infection, with the strength of the recommendation depending on the CD4 count. Here's the way I look at it:

1. If you have AIDS, if your CD4 count is less than 200, or if you have serious symptoms caused by HIV, you should start ART *immediately*. Without treatment, you're at risk for developing serious but preventable complications, some of them fatal.

2. If your CD4 count is between 200 and 500, you should start ART soon. You may feel healthy, but your immune system is already damaged. Why wait for it to get worse?

3. If your CD4 count is over 500, you should strongly consider starting ART. It may not be urgent because your risk of most HIV-related complications is low, but there may other long-term complications that can be prevented by starting ART now.

4. If you have an HIV-negative sexual partner or partners, you should start ART. Being on ART with an undetectable viral load is the most effective way to protect your partner.

Antiretroviral drugs work by interfering with one of the stages of the life cycle, and they're classified based on which stage they inhibit.

There are other reasons to start ART regardless of your CD4 count:

- *Pregnancy.* To prevent transmission to the baby (Question 76).

- *Hepatitis B.* Because you can treat both HIV and hepatitis B with the same drugs (Question 80).

- *HIV-associated nephropathy (HIVAN).* Because ART is the only effective treatment (Question 49).

- *Coronary heart disease (or high cardiac risk).* Because HIV increases your risk for heart disease (Question 47).

- *Risk of sexual transmission.* Because lowering your viral load makes you less infectious to others (Question 86).

There are only two groups of people that I don't push to start ART: **elite controllers** (people whose viral loads are undetectable without treatment), provided they have normal and stable CD4 counts, and those who aren't ready, committed, or capable of adhering to therapy.

29. What are the classes of antiretroviral drugs, and why do they matter?

HIV goes through several stages in its lifespan, beginning with its entry into a human cell and ending with the release of new virus particles into the bloodstream that then infect new cells. This is called the viral life cycle (Figure 1). Antiretroviral drugs work by interfering with one of the stages of the life cycle, and they're classified based on which stage they inhibit. Talking about **drug classes** and life cycle stages gets a little technical, but bear with me. Knowing the classes of the drugs isn't essential, but it's useful because drugs within classes often have overlapping toxicity or resistance patterns. (It's also kind of cool.) The drugs are listed by category in **Table 3**.

1. **Entry** into the CD4 cell (**entry inhibitors**). This stage has three sub-stages:

    a. **Attachment** of **gp120**, a portion of the **envelope** (the outer part of the virus) to the **CD4 receptor** on the surface of the CD4 cell. There are no approved attachment inhibitors yet, but there are some in development.

    b. Binding of coreceptors to gp120. There are two **coreceptors** (or **chemokines**) on the cell surface—**CCR5** and **CXCR4**. Maraviroc (*Selzentry*) is a drug that blocks CCR5 (**CCR5 antagonist**), and others may be developed. We don't have any drugs that block CXCR4 attachment. Before using a CCR5 inhibitor, you need a special blood test called a **tropism assay** to make sure you have purely **R5 virus** (virus that enters the cell using only the CCR5 coreceptor). If some of your virus gets in through CXCR4 (**X4 or dual/mixed [D/M] virus**), it won't be suppressed by the drug.

    c. **Fusion** (merging) of the coating of the virus with the surface of the CD4 cell, which allows the genetic material (RNA) of the virus to enter the cell. Enfuvirtide (T-20, *Fuzeon*) is an approved injectable drug that's rarely used anymore.

2. **Reverse transcription** turns viral RNA into DNA. It's called "reverse" because it's the opposite of normal transcription, which turns DNA into RNA. This process requires

gp120

The part of the envelope (outer surface) of HIV that binds to receptors on the surface of the CD4 cell, allowing entry into the cell.

Envelope

The outer surface of the HIV virus.

CD4 receptor

A protein on the surface of the CD4 cell that the virus attaches to before entering the cell.

Coreceptor (or chemokines)

Proteins on the surface of the CD4 cell and other cells that the virus binds to after attaching to the CD4 receptor but before entering the cell.

CCR5 and CXCR4

Coreceptors on the cell surface.

CCR5 antagonist

A drug that blocks CCR5.

STARTING TREATMENT

TABLE 3 Antiretroviral Agents (approved drugs in alphabetical order by drug class)

Generic Name	Brand Name	Abbreviation	Manufacturer (of brand-name version)
Nucleoside/nucleotide analog reverse transcriptase inhibitors (NRTIs)			
Abacavir	*Ziagen* or generic	ABC	ViiV Healthcare
Didanosine	*Videx, Videx EC,* or generic	ddl, ddl EC	Bristol-Myers Squibb
Emtricitabine	*Emtriva*	FTC	Gilead Sciences
Lamivudine	*Epivir* or generic	3TC	ViiV Healthcare
Stavudine	*Zerit* or generic	d4T	Bristol-Myers Squibb
Tenofovir disoproxil fumarate	*Viread*	TDF	Gilead Sciences
Zidovudine	*Retrovir* or generic	AZT, ZDV	ViiV Healthcare
Tenofovir alafenamide	Not approved*	TAF	Gilead Sciences
Non-nucleoside reverse transcriptase inhibitors (NNRTIs)			
Delavirdine	*Rescriptor*	DLV	ViiV Healthcare
Efavirenz	*Sustiva (Stocrin[†])*	EFV	Bristol-Myers Squibb (Merck & Co.[†])
Etravirine	*Intelence*	ETR	Janssen Therapeutics
Nevirapine	*Viramune, Viramune XR* or generic	NVP	Boehringer-Ingelheim
Rilpivirine	*Edurant*	RPV	Janssen Therapeutics
Doravirine	Not approved*	DOR	Merck & Co.
Protease inhibitors (PIs)			
Atazanavir	*Reyataz*	ATV	Bristol-Myers Squibb
Atazanavir/cobicistat	*Evotaz*	ATV/COBI	Bristol-Myers Squibb
Darunavir	*Prezista*	DRV	Janssen Therapeutics
Darunavir/cobicistat	*Prezcobix*	DRV/COBI	Janssen Therapeutics
Fosamprenavir	*Lexiva (Telzir[†])*	FPV	ViiV Healthcare
Indinavir	*Crixivan*	IDV	Merck & Co.
Lopinavir/ritonavir	*Kaletra (Aluvia[†])*	LPV/r	AbbVie
Nelfinavir	*Viracept*	NFV	ViiV Healthcare (Roche[†])
Ritonavir	*Norvir*	RTV	AbbVie
Saquinavir	*Invirase*	SQV	Genentech
Tipranavir	*Aptivus*	TPV	Boehringer-Ingelheim
Fusion inhibitor			
Enfuvirtide	*Fuzeon*	ENF (T20)	Genentech

Generic Name	Brand Name	Abbreviation	Manufacturer (of brand-name version)
CCR5 antagonist			
Maraviroc	*Selzentry (Celsentri[†])*	MVC	ViiV Healthcare
Integrase Inhibitors			
Raltegravir	*Isentress*	RAL	Merck & Co.
Elvitegravir	*Vitekta*	EVG	Gilead Sciences
Dolutegravir	*Tivicay*	DTG	ViiV Healthcare
Combination pills			
Abacavir/lamivudine	*Epzicom (Kivexa[†])*	ABC/3TC	ViiV Healthcare
Tenofovir/emtricitabine	*Truvada*	TDF/FTC	Gilead Sciences
Zidovudine/lamivudine	*Combivir* or generic	AZT/3TC	ViiV Healthcare
Tenofovir alafenamide/ emtricitabine	Not approved*	TAF/FTC	Gilead Sciences
Single-tablet regimens			
Abacavir/lamivudine/ zidovudine	*Trizivir*	AZT/3TC/ABC	ViiV Healthcare
Abacavir/lamivudine/ dolutegravir	*Triumeq*	ABC/3TC/DTG	ViiV Healthcare
Tenofovir/emtricitabine/ efavirenz	*Atripla*	TDF/FTC/EFV	Gilead Sciences
Tenofovir/emtricitabine/ rilpivirine	*Complera (Eviplera[†])*	TDF/FTC/RPV	Gilead Sciences
Tenofovir/emtricitabine/ elvitegravir/cobicistat	*Stribild*	TDF/FTC/EVG/ COBI	Gilead Sciences
Tenofovir alafenamide/ emtricitabine/elvitegra- vir/ cobicistat	Not approved*	TAF/FTC/EVG/COBI	Gilead Sciences
Tenofovir alafenamide/ emtricitabine/rilpivirine	Not approved*	TAF/FTC/RPV	Gilead Sciences
Tenofovir alafenamide/ emtricitabine/darunavir/ cobicistat	Not approved*	TAF/FTC/DRV/COBI	Janssen Therapeutics
Pharmacoenhancers ("boosters")			
Cobicistat	*Tybost*	COBI	Gilead Sciences

* Drugs not FDA-approved as of May 1, 2015
[†] Brand names/manufacturers in some countries outside the United States

Tropism assay

A blood test used to find out whether your virus enters the CD4 cell using the CCR5 coreceptor (R5 virus) or the CXCR4 coreceptor (X4 virus). This test is necessary before taking a CCR5 inhibitor, which should only be used with R5 virus.

R5 virus

HIV that enters the CD4 cell using the CCR5 coreceptor. This type of virus can be treated with CCR5 inhibitors.

X4 (or dual/mixed [D/M]) virus

HIV that enters the CD4 cell using the CXCR4 coreceptor. X4 virus cannot be treated with CCR5 inhibitors.

Fusion

The final stage of entry in which the envelope of the virus fuses (merges) with the membrane of the cell, allowing entry of the virus into the cells. A fusion inhibitor blocks this process.

Reverse transcription

The conversion of viral RNA into DNA by reverse transcriptase.

reverse transcriptase (**RT**), an enzyme (protein) that's brought into the cell from the virus. There are two types of reverse transcriptase inhibitors:

a. **Nucleoside analog reverse transcriptase inhibitors** (**NRTIs** or "nukes") mimic the normal building blocks of DNA. They get inserted into the growing DNA chain, but because they're not the right nucleosides, they "muck up" the process, stopping the DNA chain from being formed.

b. **Non-nucleoside reverse transcriptase inhibitors** (**NNRTIs**) stop the same process, but they do it by binding directly to the reverse transcriptase enzyme, preventing it from doing its dirty work.

3. **Integration** is the insertion of the newly created viral DNA into the human DNA in the cell's nucleus. This step requires a viral enzyme called **integrase**. **Integrase inhibitors** prevent integrase from doing its job.

4. **Protease** inhibitors (PIs) block a late stage in the viral life cycle in which proteins created from viral DNA are cleaved (cut) to create the building blocks of the new viral particles.

5. Maturation inhibitors are somewhat like protease inhibitors, but they block the cleavage of viral proteins in a different way. There is a maturation inhibitor in development.

Mike's comment:

Whether or not you understand this—I don't, except for a few random words—the good news is that the meds work if you take them the way you're supposed to.

30. How do my provider and I choose my first regimen?

Answering a question like this in a book is challenging, because my answer may be out of date by the time you read it. Things change fast as new drugs are developed and new data emerge. The Appendix lists a number of resources that can help keep you up to date, including my own interactive blog.

First, make sure you've had a baseline resistance test (Question 24) before choosing your regimen. You don't want to take a drug you're already resistant to. Besides being a waste of time and money, it could put you at risk of developing resistance to the other drugs in your regimen.

Your provider needs to know some things about you to help determine the best regimen. What other medical conditions do you have? What medications do you take? Are your kidneys and liver in good shape? What's your daily schedule like? Do you eat regular meals? Are you likely to miss doses or stop therapy? If you're a woman, is there a possibility of pregnancy?

There are also questions that you need to ask your provider, nurse, or pharmacist before you start. Should I take my meds with food or without? Does the time of day I take the meds matter? How do I get refills? What if I'm late for a dose (Question 31)? If I run out of one medication, should I still take the others? What side effects can I expect, and what should I do if I get certain side effects (Question 32)? Don't start therapy until your questions have been answered.

Reverse transcriptase (RT)

An enzyme contained within the HIV virus that can turn viral RNA into DNA so it can be inserted into the DNA of human cells. A reverse transcriptase inhibitor blocks this process.

Nucleoside analog reverse transcriptase inhibitors (NRTIs)

A class of antiretroviral drugs that blocks reverse transcription of viral RNA into DNA by mimicking nucleosides, the normal building blocks of DNA.

Non-nucleoside reverse transcriptase inhibitors (NNRTIs)

A class of antiretroviral drugs that blocks reverse transcription of viral RNA into DNA by interfering with the activity of reverse transcriptase.

Integration

The insertion of viral DNA into human DNA in the nucleus of the cell.

STARTING TREATMENT

Integrase

A viral enzyme that allows integration (insertion) of viral DNA into human DNA.

Integrase inhibitor

An antiretroviral drug that blocks this process.

Protease

A viral enzyme that cuts large viral proteins into smaller proteins, which are then used to create new virus particles. A protease inhibitor (PI) is an antiretroviral drug that blocks this process.

Adherence (or compliance)

The term used to refer to a patient's behavior with respect to following treatment recommendations, including taking medications, keeping medical appointments, etc.

HLA B*5701

A blood test used to predict the likelihood of the abacavir hypersensitivity reaction (HSR). If the test is positive, you shouldn't take abacavir. If it's negative, you're extremely unlikely to develop HSR.

Table 4 lists the advantages and disadvantages of the various drugs, combination pills, and single-tablet regimens. The recommended starting regimens all include either a non-nucleoside reverse transcriptase inhibitor (NNRTI), a protease inhibitor (PI), or an integrase inhibitor (sometimes abbreviated INSTI for "integrase strand transfer inhibitor" because "II" would be too weird). These agents are almost always used in combination with two nucleoside analog reverse transcriptase inhibitors (NRTIs), which are sometimes called the "nuke backbone." The two recommended backbones are tenofovir/emtricitabine (available as *Truvada*) and abacavir/lamivudine (available in generic form or as *Epzicom* or *Kivexa*, depending on what country you live in.) The decision about whether to use a tenofovir- or abacavir-based regimen depends on several factors. Tenofovir can sometimes cause kidney damage, and there is a greater loss of bone density with tenofovir than with other NRTIs. There is controversy about whether abacavir increases the risk of heart attack, which is mainly an issue for people who have a lot of cardiac risk factors already. You must get an **HLA B*5701** test before taking any regimen containing abacavir (*Ziagen, Epivir, Trizivir, Triumeq*), because it can cause a serious hypersensitivity reaction in those who test positive. In people with viral loads above 100,000, *Epzicom* was less effective than *Truvada* in combination with some third agents, but that doesn't apply when it's combined with dolutegravir (usually in the form of *Triumeq*).

As for third agents, I'll start with the INSTIs. They're quickly becoming a favorite way to start based on their outstanding safety and tolerability in **clinical trials**, with effectiveness that's at least as good as the PIs or NNRTIs, and sometimes better. In fact, four of the five initial regimens recommended in U.S. government treatment guidelines include INSTIs. Raltegravir (*Isentress*) was the first INSTI, and although it's an excellent drug, it does require twice-daily dosing and is not available in a single-tablet regimen (STR). A once-daily form is being studied. Raltegravir has almost no drug interactions, an advantage for some people who are taking many other medications. *Stribild* is an STR that combines the INSTI elvitegravir with cobicistat, a drug that boosts elvitegravir levels, and the nuke backbone of tenofovir/lamivudine. It's well tolerated and effective, but cobicistat has drug interactions that are similar to those of ritonavir (*Norvir*) (Question 34). Elvitegravir and cobicistat are both available as stand-alone products (*Vitekta* and *Tybost*, respectively), but they're used much less often than *Stribild*. Dolutegravir (*Tivicay*) is the newest INSTI. It appears to have a somewhat higher barrier to resistance than the others. It can be prescribed with *Truvada* or as an STR with abacavir and lamivudine (*Triumeq*). It has a few more drug interactions than raltegravir, but not many.

Among the NNRTIs, efavirenz (*Sustiva*, and in combination with tenofovir/emtricitabine as *Atripla*) has been the favored NNRTI for years because of its long-term safety and effectiveness in many clinical trials. Unfortunately, it causes "neuropsychiatric" side effects—dizziness, vivid dreams, nightmares, fuzzy thinking, and "brain fog"—during the first few days or weeks (Question 52). Some side effects can be longer lasting, including depression. As a result, it's becoming less popular than it used to be, given all the other regimens that don't take getting used to. Rilpivirine (*Edurant*, and in combination with tenofovir/emtricitabine as *Complera* or *Eviplera*, depending on the country you live in) is much better tolerated, but it has to be taken with a meal, and you can't take it with drugs such as proton pump inhibitors that are used to treat heartburn, reflux, and ulcers.

Clinical trial

A study in which a treatment for a medical condition is tested in human volunteers to determine the safety and/or effectiveness of the treatment. In the case of HIV, this could include the study of investigational or approved drugs. See Glossary for more information.

STARTING TREATMENT

Table 4 Advantages and Disadvantages of Antiretroviral Drugs and Regimens for Initial Therapy

Drug/ Regimen	Forms and Brand Names	Advantages	Disadvantages
Recommended initial regimens all consist of two NRTIs (the "backbone") plus a third agent.			
Nucleoside analog reverse transcriptase inhibitor "backbones" (to be combined with third agent)			
Tenofovir/ emtricitabine (TDF/FTC)	*Truvada* (and part of *Atripla, Complera,* and *Stribild*)	• The recommended NRTI backbone in combination with most third agents. • 3 single-tablet regimens (STRs) available: *Atripla, Complera,* and *Stribild* • Both drugs active against hepatitis B	• Can cause kidney toxicity (monitor creatinine and urinalysis) • Causes more loss of bone density than other drugs
Abacavir/ lamivudine (ABC/3TC)	*Epzicom, Kivexa* (and part of *Trizivir* and *Triumeq*)	• No kidney toxicity • Available in a guidelines-recommended STR with DTG (*Triumeq*)	• Must pre-test with HLA B*5701 to avoid ABC hypersensitivity reaction • Less effective than TDF/ FTC when combined with EFV or ATV/r in people with viral loads above 100,000 • May increase risk of heart attack (controversial)
Didanosine (ddI)	*Videx, Videx EC,* or generic	• None	• Not recommended
Stavudine (d4T)	*Zerit, Zerit XR,* or generic	• None	• Not recommended
Zidovudine (ZDV, AZT)	*Retrovir* or generic (and part of *Combivir, Trizivir*)	• Safe in pregnancy	• Not recommended
THIRD AGENTS			
Non-nucleoside reverse transcriptase inhibitors			
Efavirenz (EFV)	*Sustiva* (and part of *Atripla*)	• Extensively studied • STR available (*Atripla*) • Remains in blood for a long time: "forgiving" of missed doses	• Can cause neurologic or psychiatric side effects, especially in the first few weeks, but long-term effects also occur

Drug/ Regimen	Forms and Brand Names	Advantages	Disadvantages
Efavirenz (EFV) (*continued*)		• See TDF advantages (for *Atripla*)	• Can cause rash • Resistance common if treatment fails • May cause birth defects if given to pregnant women during first trimester • Less CD4 increase than with other third agents (PIs, INSTIs) • See TDF disadvantages (for *Atripla*) • Now classified as an alternative regimen (DHHS guidelines)
Rilpivirine (RPV)	*Edurant* (and part of *Complera, Eviplera*)	• STR available (*Complera*) • Better tolerated than *Sustiva, Atripla* (less rash, neurologic side effects, and effect on lipids)	• Must be taken with a meal • Can't be taken with proton pump inhibitors, drugs used to treat reflux and ulcers • Resistance common if treatment fails • Failure may cause cross-resistance to ETR • Classified as alternative regimen in DHHS guidelines, only if viral load below 100,000 and CD4 above 200
Delavirdine (DLV)	*Rescriptor*	• None	• Not recommended
Nevirapine (NVP)	*Viramune, Viramune XR,* or generic	• Well tolerated • Safest NNRTI in pregnancy • Generic form available	• Not recommended for initial therapy (U.S. guidelines) • Can cause severe liver toxicity or skin rash during first few weeks, especially in women with pre-treatment CD4 counts above 250 or men with counts above 400 • Resistance common if treatment fails

(continues)

Table 4 Advantages and Disadvantages of Antiretroviral Drugs and Regimens for Initial Therapy (continued)

Drug/ Regimen	Forms and Brand Names	Advantages	Disadvantages
THIRD AGENTS			
Protease Inhibitors (PIs)			
Atazanavir/ritonavir (ATV/r), atazanavir/ cobicistat (ATV/cobi), or atazanavir (ATV)	*Reyataz/Norvir, Evotaz,* or *Reyataz*	• The best PI if boosting not possible (boosting required if taken with TDF) • Resistance unlikely with failure (when boosted)	• Can cause jaundice • Should be taken with food • Should not be taken with proton pump inhibitors (drugs used to treat reflux and ulcers) • More GI side effects than DRV • Can cause kidney stones, gallstones, or kidney toxicity (uncommon) • Now classified as an alternative regimen (DHHS guidelines)
Darunavir/ ritonavir (DRV/r) or darunavir/ cobicistat (DRV/cobi)	*Prezista/Norvir* or *Prezcobix*	• The best tolerated PI • Resistance unlikely with failure • With ritonavir boosting, the only recommended PI-based regimen (DHHS guidelines)	• Should be taken with food • Can cause rash
Lopinavir/ritonavir (LPV/r)	*Kaletra, Aluvia*	• Best studied PI in pregnant women • Resistance unlikely with failure	• No longer recommended for initial therapy (U.S. guidelines) • More GI side effects than ATV or DRV • Affects cholesterol and triglycerides more than ATV or DRV
Fosamprenavir (FPV)	*Lexiva*	• Can be given unboosted	• No longer recommended for initial therapy

Drug/ Regimen	Forms and Brand Names	Advantages	Disadvantages
Indinavir (IDV)	*Crixivan*	• None	• Not recommended
Nelfinavir (NFV)	*Viracept*	• None	• Not recommended
Ritonavir (RTV)	*Norvir*	• Used only as low-dose booster for other PIs	• Should not be used at full dose to treat HIV infection
Saquinavir (SQV)	*Invirase*	• None	• Not recommended
Integrase Inhibitors			
Raltegravir (RAL)	*Isentress*	• Few side effects • Few drug interactions • With *Truvada*, a recommended regimen (DHHS guidelines)	• Twice-daily dosing
Elvitegravir (EVG)	*Vitekta* or part of *Stribild*	• See TDF advantages • Part of STR • Better tolerated than EFV or PIs • *Stribild* is a recommended regimen (DHHS guidelines)	• See TDF disadvantages • COBI drug interactions similar to RTV • COBI causes increase in creatinine, giving *appearance* of decreased kidney function. Avoid if kidney function poor.
Dolutegravir (DTG)	*Tivicay* or part of *Triumeq*	• Few side effects • Few drug interactions • Higher barrier to resistance than RAL or EVG • See ABC advantages (for *Triumeq*) • *Triumeq* is the only non-TDF-containing STR • *Tivicay/Truvada* or Triumeq are recommended regimens (DHHS guidelines)	• See ABC disadvantages (for *Triumeq*)

Nevirapine (*Viramune*) has fallen out of favor, mainly because it can have severe early side effects in people who start therapy with high CD4 counts. Delavirdine (*Rescriptor*) is no longer recommended, and etravirine (*Intelence*) is generally not used for initial therapy.

Boosted protease inhibitors

These combine a protease inhibitor (PI) with cobicistat or with a low dose of ritonavir (*Norvir*), another PI that is used only to increase drug levels and prolong the half-life of other PIs.

PIs today are virtually always **boosted**, either with low doses of ritonavir (*Norvir*), a PI that's much too toxic to use at full dose, or with cobicistat. These pharmacoenhancers or "boosters" increase drug levels of the PIs, increasing their potency and allowing you to take them less often or with fewer pills. A clear advantage of boosted PI regimens is that they're virtually resistance-proof, making them ideal for people who aren't good at taking medications faithfully. The favored PI for initial therapy is now darunavir (*Prezista*). It is available in combination with cobicistat: *Prezcobix*, so it's no longer necessary to take separate doses of *Norvir*. Another commonly used PI is atazanavir (*Reyataz*), which is also available as *Evotaz*, a combination with cobicistat. There's little reason to use any of the older PIs anymore.

By the time you read this, a new form of tenofovir—tenofovir alafenamide (TAF)—may have been approved in combination pills that contain other drugs. Compared to tenofovir DF, the form we've been using for many years, TAF appears to be safer for kidneys and to have virtually no effect on bone density. My expectation is that TAF will quickly replace TDF, though much of that will depend on price and the whims of the insurance companies and other third-party payers.

31. Why is adherence so important?

Adherence (or compliance) is the word we use to describe your ability to "stick to" treatment recommendations, including taking medications and keeping clinic appointments. Adherence is important for any medical treatment, but it's *especially* important for HIV infection because of the risk of drug resistance. If you were non-adherent with your blood pressure medications, you might damage your heart, kidneys, or vision, but the drugs would still work once you started taking them properly. No matter how bad you are at keeping diabetes under control, insulin will work when it's taken. In contrast, HIV is a living organism whose sole reason for living is to replicate (reproduce itself). ART stops that replication. Missed doses and interruptions in treatment allow drug levels to fall. If they fall low enough, the virus starts replicating again. When it does, resistant mutants—virus particles that can replicate in the presence of drugs—have an advantage over the drug-sensitive strains. They can eventually replace the non-resistant (wild-type) virus as the dominant viral strain.

For a particularly vivid analogy that you won't soon forget, imagine a can full of the creatures from your nightmares: rats, cockroaches, spiders, or snakes—your choice. If you keep the lid on the can, the critters can't get out. But if you leave the lid ajar, the strongest will escape. They'll hook up with the other strong escapees, breeding super-creatures that you won't want to have around. Adherence to ART is the lid on the can. Keep it tightly closed!

Adherence (or compliance)

The term used to refer to a patient's behavior with respect to following treatment recommendations, including taking medications, keeping medical appointments, etc.

STARTING TREATMENT

Studies show that your ability to adhere to therapy has little to do with your race, sex, education level, or socio-economic status. Things that *do* affect adherence are mental illness (including depression), drug or alcohol abuse, memory problems, and a chaotic lifestyle. If any of those issues apply to you, address them before starting therapy (Part 13). I also find that my patients are more likely to adhere if they understand why they're on treatment, why adherence is important, and if they participated in the decision to start treatment. Finally, it helps to have what is called "self-efficacy": the confidence that you have the ability to affect your future by completing actions you take in the present.

Fortunately, adherence is easier now because the available regimens are better tolerated, are usually taken just once day, and typically consist of 1–2 pills. The newer drugs have longer **half-lives** than the older drugs, which means they last a long time in the blood. That gives you more "wiggle room" in the timing of doses. But missing doses or interrupting treatment is still risky, especially with NNRTIs and some INSTIs, because it only takes a single mutation to get high-level resistance. If you're worried about your ability to adhere to therapy, talk to your provider, nurse, or pharmacist before you start therapy. Many HIV clinics have programs that can help with adherence.

Half-life

The amount of time it takes for the blood levels of a drug to decline by 50% after the last dose. Drugs with longer half-lives remain in the blood longer and can be taken less often.

Here are a few tips to help you adhere:

1. Get a pillbox from the pharmacy—one that has labeled compartments for each day and dose. Put your pills in it each week, even if you're only taking one pill per day. You'll never have to wonder whether you took your pills or not—if they're still in the box, you didn't.

2. Link your doses to something else you do *every* day—eating a meal, brushing your teeth, or making coffee. If you have a cup of coffee every morning, put your pills beside the coffee maker so you see them when you reach for your morning cup.

3. Always check your medication supply and order your refills in advance—don't run out on weekends or holidays. If you're using a mail-order pharmacy, you have to plan even further ahead.

4. Talk to your provider or pharmacist about what to do if you forget a dose. With most HIV drugs, it's OK to take them as soon as you remember, or even to double the next dose, but I wouldn't suggest doubling the dose of efavirenz (*Sustiva, Atripla*) because of the side effects you're likely to experience.

My patients who do best are the ones who are a little obsessive-compulsive about taking their medications. When I ask, "How many doses have you missed since I saw you last?" they look at me as if I'd asked them about the last time they'd clubbed a group of baby seals.

Mike's comments:

I talk sternly to myself about the importance of taking my medicine as prescribed. My goal is to never miss a dose. I NEVER consult my mood when it's time to take my medicine. There is no good enough reason to miss a dose, and besides, the virus isn't reasonable. The tools I use are a pillbox and good, healthy, empowering fear. The fear reminds me why I need to take meds, and the pillbox tells me whether or not I've taken them. Taking every dose, as prescribed, gives me peace of mind—I'm doing what I need to do to help myself. And it only takes a minute or two a day. I now take my meds once a day (down from three times a day), and I also take medicine for high cholesterol, osteoporosis, and herpes. I've been taking meds for over 10 years now, so I figure I've taken around 10,000 doses. While I never forget that I need to take medication, remembering each dose as a discrete event is impossible. The pillbox is a fail-safe tool.

32. What if I have side effects?

Side effects

Undesirable effects of a medication or treatment that are noticeable to the person being treated.

Toxicity

Damage to the body caused by a drug or other substance.

I'll been using two terms—**side effects** and **toxicity**, which are not always the same thing. Side effects make your life unpleasant, but they don't always mean that the drugs are hurting you (for example, nervous system side effects from efavirenz, discussed in Question 52). On the other hand, you may feel fine even though you're taking a drug that's causing toxicity (for example, high cholesterol from some PIs, Question 43). Finally, you may have a side effect that's also a toxicity, such as painful feet caused by nerve damage from stavudine (Questions 45 and 52).

Pancreatitis

Inflammation of the pancreas, resulting in abdominal pain, loss of appetite, nausea, and vomiting. Can be fatal.

Hypersensitivity reactions (HSRs)

Reactions, often allergic, to a medication or other substance.

Because you'll be starting at least three new medications at once, it's not unusual to experience side effects. Side effects and toxicities of specific drugs are discussed in Part 8. Some side effects, such as the nervous system side effects of efavirenz or upset stomach with zidovudine, are temporary. Others are chronic but manageable, such as loose stools with PIs. Some can be acute and serious, such as **pancreatitis** with didanosine or **hypersensitivity reactions** (**HSRs**) with abacavir or nevirapine. Other side effects can get worse with continued use (nerve damage with stavudine) or can cause a risk of long-term problems (high cholesterol or blood sugar due to PIs, which increase the risk of heart disease). Fortunately, *none* of the drugs I've just mentioned is a recommended drug that's commonly used today.

Today's drugs are a lot easier to put up with than the older ones.

Starting therapy is sometimes a trial-and-error process. You may end up on a different combination than the one you started on. Substituting one drug for another because of side effects is fine, and is much safer than stopping completely and starting over later, which can increase the risk of resistance. When starting your first regimen, it's important to know how to contact your provider if you have unexpected side effects or side effects that you can't put up with until your next visit.

Mike's comment:

I started taking HIV meds nearly 20 years ago, and I can tell you that the side effects of the newer meds I'm on now are zilch. There are no associated toxicities either, at least so far. A friend of mine, who was supposed to start taking meds, filled his prescriptions and then postponed starting for a few months, afraid he would feel sick. When he finally started, he sheepishly admitted to me that he had no side effects at all.

33. How should my treatment be monitored?

Once you start ART, it's important to get lab tests done frequently—usually every month or so at the beginning. The purpose of monitoring is to make sure you're responding to the medications appropriately and not developing toxicity.

The best measure of response to therapy is your viral load. It should decrease at least tenfold in the first month, which means that if it started out at 100,000, it should be well below 10,000. Your viral load should then continue to fall until it becomes undetectable (less than 20), usually within 4–6 months. Integrase inhibitors will lower the viral load much faster—often within 1–2 months. That doesn't necessarily make them better, but it's still gratifying. I generally check the viral load every 4–6 weeks until it becomes undetectable, then every 3–4 months after that. In my patients who have had undetectable viral loads for many years, I often switch to a 6-month schedule.

The CD4 count will also increase on therapy, but the amount of increase is impossible to predict. Starting with a low CD4 count, having a low baseline viral load, having hepatitis C, or being older can all blunt the CD4 response to therapy. In the past, we always ordered a CD4 count every time we checked the viral load, but that's no longer recommended because the viral load is so much more important. Once your viral load is undetectable and your CD4 count is high and stable, it becomes an optional test.

We look for drug toxicity with standard blood tests. The complete blood count (CBC) measures the red and white blood cell counts and the platelet count. The only antiretroviral medication that's likely to affect these counts is zidovudine (AZT), which can cause **anemia** (low red blood cell count). A comprehensive chemistry panel includes measurements of kidney function, liver health, and blood sugar. A urinalysis should be checked twice a year if you're taking a regimen that includes tenofovir (*Viread, Truvada, Complera, Atripla, Stribild*). You should get a fasting lipid panel and blood sugar at least once a year, especially if you're taking medications that have metabolic side effects.

Starting therapy is sometimes a trial-and-error process. You may end up on a different combination than the one you started on. Substituting one drug for another because of side effects is fine.

Anemia

A deficiency of red blood cells, usually diagnosed by a low hemoglobin or hematocrit on a complete blood count.

34. Can my HIV drugs interact with other medications?

They sure can, which is why you should always carry a list of all of the medicines you're taking, and show the list to other providers who are treating you. The PIs, NNRTIs, cobicistat, and CCR5 antagonist are the drugs most likely to interact with other medications, and also with each other. There are few interactions with NRTIs, fusion inhibitors, raltegravir, and dolutegravir. Listing all drug interactions here would be impossible, but I'll make a few points about interactions that are especially common and important:

- *Statins.* The levels of the **statins** (drugs that lower cholesterol) can be increased by ritonavir (*Norvir*) and cobicistat (*Tybost, Prezcobix, Evotaz*), causing muscle breakdown and kidney failure. Some, such as simvastatin (*Zocor*) and lovastatin (*Mevacor*), should *never* be used with PIs or cobicistat. Others, such as atorvastatin (*Lipitor*), pravastatin (*Pravachol*), and rosuvastatin (*Crestor*), can generally be used at low doses, though pravastatin—a weaker statin—should be avoided with darunavir (*Prezista, Prezcobix*). A newer agent, pitavastatin (*Livalo*), has no important drug interactions.

- *Birth control pills.* PIs, NNRTIs, and cobicistat can lower drug levels, making them less effective, so you may need to use another method of birth control if you're taking one of these drugs.

- *Rifampin.* **Rifampin** is a drug used to treat tuberculosis and some bacterial infections. It affects the levels of most PIs and NNRTIs. It shouldn't be taken with any PI or NNRTI except efavirenz. If you're using nevirapine or PIs, rifabutin can be used as an alternative.

STARTING TREATMENT

Statins
The common name for HMG CoA reductase inhibitors, drugs that lower cholesterol.

Carry a list of all of the medicines you're taking, and show that list to other providers who are treating you.

Rifampin
A drug used to treat tuberculosis and some other bacterial infections.

- *Steroid sprays.* PIs and cobicistat can increase steroid levels with fluticasone, a common ingredient in nasal sprays or inhalers (*Flonase, Advair, Flovent*). Use alternatives if possible. This interaction is also a problem with steroids that are injected into joints to treat pain.

- *Narcotics.* Methadone levels are decreased by some NNRTIs and PIs, which can cause withdrawal. Fentanyl levels can be increased, resulting in overdose.

- *Proton pump inhibitors* (PPIs)*. These drugs, used to treat acid reflux and ulcers, should generally not be used with atazanavir (*Reyataz, Evotaz*) or rilpivirine (*Edurant, Complera, Eviplera*), because the PPIs can lower the HIV drugs' absorption so that you get less than the dose you need. If you have to take a PPI with one of these drugs, it should be at the lowest dose and with careful dose separation. Other drugs that lower stomach acid, such as antacids and H2-blockers,† also require dose separation.

- *Calcium channel blockers.*‡ PIs and cobicistat can increase the levels of these drugs, used to treat high blood pressure, which can increase the risk of side effects.

- *Seizure medications.* It's important to check drug levels of a number of seizure medications if you're on ART to make sure you're getting the right dose. Some seizure medications can lower drug levels of some HIV drugs. Levetiracetam (*Keppra*) is a good

---

*PPIs: Omeprazole (*Prilosec*), esomeprazole (*Nexium*), pantoprazole (*Protonix*), lansoprazole (*Prevacid*), and rabeprazole (*Aciphex*).

†H2-blockers: Ranitidine (*Zantac*), cimetidine (*Tagamet*), and famotidine (*Pepcid*).

‡Calcium channel blockers: Nifedipine (*Adalat, Procardia*), verapamil (*Calan*), and diltiazem (*Cardizem, Tiazac,* and others).

choice if you need a seizure medication, because it doesn't interact with HIV drugs.

- *Alternative therapies.* Don't forget that many **complementary medicine** and **alternative medicine** therapies, such as herbal supplements, are *drugs* from the body's point of view and can interact with prescribed medications (Questions 41 and 91).

This is *not* a complete list. When in doubt, ask your provider or pharmacist.

Complementary medicine

The use of a non-standard medical treatment in addition to standard therapy.

Alternative medicine

The use of a non-standard medical treatment in place of standard therapy.

STARTING TREATMENT

PART SEVEN

Staying on Therapy

How long will therapy last?

Can therapy ever be stopped?

How will I know if my therapy stops working?

More…

35. How long will therapy last?

If you're taking well chosen therapy and you're not missing doses, your first regimen can last as long as you do,
or until something better comes along. In the bad old
days, we'd start treatment with zidovudine (AZT),
would see a rise in CD4 count that might last for a
year or two if we were lucky, but then things would
start to get worse. We'd try another NRTI or a combination of two NRTIs, and the benefit would be even
shorter. Because we weren't able to fully suppress the
viral load with NRTIs, resistance began evolving from
the moment they were started. The inevitable result of
therapy was resistance to the drug that was being taken
and **cross-resistance** to other drugs in the same class.

Things changed completely in the mid-1990s with the
availability of PIs, NNRTIs, and the concept of combination therapy, not just because we started using three
drugs, but because we went from merely lowering viral
replication to stopping it altogether. Now that we can
keep the virus from replicating, we can stop mutations
from occurring and prevent resistance. It's theoretically
possible for the benefits of a single ART regimen to be
permanent—as long as you continue to take it faithfully.

Some researchers believe that the virus is replicating at
very low levels, even when the viral load is undetectable.
If they're right, then resistance could emerge eventually,
though it might take decades. Others believe that there
is no replication and point to studies showing that the
virus of highly adherent patients after many years on
ART is identical to the one they started with, with no
evolution of resistance.

My patients don't fail therapy without a reason. Those
who fail are almost always non-adherent. When failure

Cross-resistance

Resistance to one drug that results in resistance to other drugs, usually in the same class.

---

*It's theoreti-
cally possible
for the benefits
of a single
ART regimen
to be perma-
nent as long
as you con-
tinue to take it
faithfully.*

does occur, we have plenty of good treatment options. I'm confident that if taken correctly, ART will last for a lifetime.

36. Can therapy ever be stopped?

It can, but it's always a bad idea. You should assume that once you start ART, you're in it for the long haul. We used to hear a lot about **treatment interruption** (**drug holidays** or **structured treatment interruptions**). Many patients were tired of side effects and wanted a break. Researchers thought that occasional structured treatment interruptions might allow people to recover from drug toxicity without harm, provided the CD4 count stayed in a safe zone.

That approach turned out to be very wrong. A large clinical trial comparing intermittent versus continuous therapy was stopped early because people who interrupted therapy were more likely to die or have serious complications than those who remained on therapy, even if they kept their CD4 counts above 250. In short, the concept of treatment interruption as a deliberate strategy quickly became dead in the water.

That doesn't mean you can't stop treatment if you absolutely have to. We sometimes have to stop therapy in people who develop serious side effects or who are too sick to take medications, but those are exceptional cases. Fortunately, now that ART has improved, staying on therapy is much easier than it used to be. Be aware that stopping NNRTI-containing regimens can be especially risky. The long half-life of drugs like efavirenz, rilpivirine, and nevirapine means that the drugs hang around for a long time—sometimes weeks after your last dose, and long after the other drugs in the regimen have

Treatment interruption

Stopping antiretroviral therapy. No longer in vogue.

Drug holiday

An old term for an interruption in therapy, usually when the decision was made by the patient.

Structured treatment interruption

An old term for an interruption in therapy that was approved by the provider.

You should assume that once you start therapy, you're in it for the long haul.

disappeared. That's a problem, because it leaves them vulnerable to resistance, and resistance to these drugs requires just a single mutation. If you should ever have to stop taking an NNRTI-based regimen, talk to your provider about safer ways to do it.

37. How will I know if my therapy stops working?

You can't tell whether therapy is working based on how you feel, or what your CD4 count is. The *only* way to know is to measure the viral load, which is always the best indicator of treatment success and failure (Question 23). Your viral load should be undetectable within 4 to 6 months of starting therapy. If your viral load doesn't decrease the way it's supposed to, or if it becomes detectable after having been undetectable, this *may* be a sign of treatment failure.

No lab test is perfect. A viral load can be detectable in people who aren't failing, often just because lab tests aren't 100 percent accurate. If you're taking your medications faithfully and you have a viral load that's detectable but low, don't panic. It's probably just a "blip"—a single detectable viral load that generally means nothing (Question 23). The only way to tell the difference between a blip and early failure is to repeat the viral load. If its falls back to undetectable levels, then it was a blip and you should forget about it. We generally get concerned only if the viral load is repeatedly above 200.

If the viral load remains detectable or is rising, there may be a problem. This should be taken seriously—even when everything else is going great—because it could mean that you're developing resistance. We can measure resistance when the viral load is above 500 to 1,000. The new *GenoSure Archive* test can measure resistance when the viral load is low or undetectable (Question 24).

The CD4 count is a lousy measure of treatment failure (Question 22). If your viral load is undetectable but your CD4 response is disappointing, changing medications won't make a difference. The best approach is to keep your viral load undetectable, and let the CD4 count do what it will do. In a person with an undetectable viral load, we know of no way to increase the CD4 count in a way that makes a meaningful clinical difference.

38. What if my virus becomes resistant to the medications?

Resistance can be the *result* of treatment failure (when you're not taking your medications properly) or it can be the *cause* of failure (when you already have resistance before you start). Resistance can occur whenever the virus is able to replicate despite the use of antiretroviral medications. Fortunately, resistance is no longer the inevitable result of ART, as it was in the bad old days. Studies show that people who take their medications faithfully rarely develop resistance.

The best way to deal with resistance is not to let it happen. If you're about to start therapy for the first time, get a resistance test to make sure your virus is susceptible to the regimen. Once you start, take every dose and keep your viral load suppressed. If you follow those two rules, you'll probably never have to read the rest of this answer.

But, to paraphrase an oft-repeated maxim, "resistance happens." When it does, I've got two more rules: (1) Act

Studies show that people who take their medications faithfully rarely develop resistance. The best way to deal with resistance is not to let it happen in the first place.

fast. Continuing a failing regimen allows more mutations and resistance to occur. (2) Get data. Resistance testing tells you which drugs your virus is resistant to and which will still work (Question 24).

We now have a lot of drugs in different classes and with different resistance profiles. If you develop resistance on your first combination, you'll still have plenty of good options. But those options might not be quite as easy or as well tolerated as the first, so make the first one last!

39. Are new drugs being developed?

Since the approval of zidovudine (AZT, *Retrovir*) in 1987, there has been a steady increase in the number of new antiretroviral agents. The first drugs were NRTIs. Two other classes, PIs and NNRTIs, were introduced in the mid-1990s. Then came enfuvirtide (T20, *Fuzeon*), a fusion inhibitor and the first entry inhibitor. 2007 was a breakthrough year, with the introduction of maraviroc (*Selzentry*), the first CCR5 antagonist; raltegravir (*Isentress*), the first INSTI; and etravirine (*Intelence*), a new "second-generation" NNRTI (Question 29). More breakthroughs followed: 2011 saw the approval of rilpivirine (*Edurant*), a new NNRTI, as well as *Complera*, a single-tablet regimen that contains rilpivirine, tenofovir, and emtricitabine. *Stribild*, the first single-tablet INSTI-containing regimen, was approved in 2012; the next year saw the approval of dolutegravir (*Tivicay*), followed in 2014 by *Triumeq*, another single-tablet INSTI regimen. There are additional entry inhibitors, NRTIs, NNRTIs, and INSTIs being developed.

The costs of bringing a new drug to market are enormous. For a drug to make it that far, it has to have a reason to exist. New drugs tend to fall into one of two categories: They either work when others don't because of a unique mechanism of action or resistance profile, or they're more convenient or less toxic than existing drugs. In addition, clinical studies must show that the drug is well absorbed, achieves adequate drug levels, suppresses viral load, and is active and safe. A lot of things can go wrong along the way, and not all drug candidates make it to the finish line.

At some point in the near future, drug companies may decide that the current therapies for HIV infection are good enough, that the competition is too stiff, and that there's no longer a financial incentive to develop new agents. That hasn't happened yet, but the pace of drug development has slowed, especially for drugs used to treat resistant virus, because there are so few people now with hard-to-treat virus. Don't assume there will always be new drugs to bail you out if you fail multiple regimens. Make your current regimen last by taking it as prescribed.

40. What if I decide not to take medications?

Virtually all HIV-positive people need treatment. I sometimes hear people say they want to fight their HIV the "natural way" instead of taking "toxic chemicals." People who talk like that are too young to remember the devastation that AIDS caused during the bad years, and they're unaware of the devastation that it's still causing in parts of the world that can't afford effective therapy. They forget that "natural" doesn't necessarily mean healthy. After all, HIV is completely "natural," and it's killing millions. In contrast, those "toxic chemicals" that we doctors love to dish out have saved countless lives and represent one of the great medical miracles of the 20th century.

Although almost everyone with HIV infection will benefit from ART, not everyone *needs* to be on therapy immediately. Question 28 talks about when treatment is urgent and when it's not. People with high CD4 counts and low viral loads could choose to be monitored without medications, but it's hard for me to imagine why anyone would want to live with a toxic, replicating, infectious virus that causes chronic inflammation and immune activation with possible downstream consequences and that puts sexual partners at risk, when the alternative is to take one or two pills every day. Elite controllers—people with undetectable viral loads who have normal and stable CD4 counts without ART—are the only people who may not benefit from ART (though even *that's* controversial). But elite controllers make up a tiny fraction of HIV-positive people, and they're the way they are because of their own genetic make-up, not because of their lifestyle, diet, herbal supplements, meditation regimen, or anything else they have control over.

We're in the fourth decade of the AIDS epidemic, and we know more than we care to know about the slow, painful death that results from untreated HIV infection. I had many patients in the 1980s and 1990s who meditated, took herbal supplements, ate healthy diets, saw faith healers, visualized their virus disappearing while holding crystals—and guess what? They died anyway. Why go back to the 1980s when you live in the 21st century? Take advantage of what medical science has to offer, and save your life!

41. Should I take complementary or alternative therapies?

Complementary and alternative medicine (CAM) is the term used to describe non-standard therapies. Complementary medicine is the use of non-standard therapy *in addition to* standard therapy; alternative medicine is the use of non-standard therapy *instead of* standard therapy. One problem with non-standard therapies is that there usually isn't enough evidence to make them standard. That doesn't mean they don't work. Natural therapies can *become* standard. There are also examples of natural substances that are very bad for you. (Socrates didn't take hemlock for his health!)

Research into the safety and benefits of CAM *is* being conducted. In fact, the National Center for Complementary and Alternative Medicine, which is part of the **National Institutes of Health (NIH)**, now gives grants for this kind of research. In some cases, the research supports the claims made about these substances; in other cases, it doesn't. So far, there have been no alternative therapies for HIV infection that have come close to matching the benefits of ART.

Another problem with CAM is that it often involves taking substances that can interact with ART drugs. Those who think of herbs as cuddly, benign, natural substances don't like to hear them called "drugs," but let's face it—if they weren't drugs, there would be no point in taking them. Antiretroviral medications interact with lots of other drugs, and we now know they can interact with herbal medications, too. The best studied example is St. John's wort, which lowers PI levels, allowing the virus to replicate and develop resistance.

> **STAYING ON THERAPY**

> **Complementary and alternative medicine (CAM)**
> Medical products or treatments that are not standard of care.

> **National Institutes of Health (NIH)**
> An agency of the federal government (under the Department of Health and Human Services) responsible for conducting and funding medical research.

> *So far, there have been no alternative therapies for HIV infection that have come close to matching the benefits of ART.*

Unfortunately, few of the many CAM therapies have been tested for interactions with HIV drugs.

When I bring up the lack of research, my CAM-supporting patients and friends tell me the tests aren't done because there's no profit in it for the big bad drug companies. But, in fact, the supplement industry is making a *fortune*. It has powerful friends in Congress who fight all attempts at regulation. If they're not studying the safety or efficacy of their products, it's because they're already doing just fine as it is without any data.

My advice: Follow the evidence. Don't be like my patient who was skeptical about every treatment I suggested, but who swallowed everything the high school drop-out at the local health food store told him to buy. Be skeptical about *everything*. Whether you're thinking of taking a prescription drug or an herb, first ask, "What's the evidence that this will help me and not hurt me?" And when you're looking for that evidence, don't be like the current anti-vaxxers, HIV denialists, and "creation scientists," who define "research" as a Google search for opinions that match their own. Use credible sources, like AIDS.gov, AIDSinfo.nih.gov, the Centers for Disease Control and Prevention website, and *of course* my own blog (www.hivforum.tumblr.com). Some of the best resources are included in the Appendix at the end of this book for you to use as a starting point.

42. What is immune-based therapy?

Immune-based therapy is treatment designed to restore the immune system or to improve its ability to fight HIV infection. It's clear that we're never going to cure HIV infection just by keeping the viral load undetectable with ART. The virus inserts its DNA into human cells, where it remains forever, waiting until treatment is stopped to create new virus particles. Our drugs work *only* on replicating virus; they have no activity against viral DNA that's hiding out in resting CD4 cells.

Theoretically, we could cure HIV infection if we could activate all resting CD4 cells and wake up the sleeping virus using "**latency**-reversing agents," allowing ART to do its thing against the activated virus. There are two problems with this approach. First, unless you activate *every* resting CD4 cell in the body, you'll still have latent virus and be no closer to a cure than you were before. Second, resting CD4 cells aren't the only reservoirs for latent HIV, but some of the proposed treatments may activate only CD4 cells.

Another immune-based approach is therapeutic vaccination. The idea here is not to eradicate HIV, but to stimulate the immune system to fight it better. A successful **therapeutic vaccine** might delay the need for ART or turn more people into elite controllers. There are vaccines being studied, but this is still an experimental approach that probably won't be put into practice any time soon.

Immune-based therapy has clearly lagged behind antiviral therapy, but that doesn't mean it doesn't have a future. Maybe I'll have better news in the next edition of this book. (I know, I know...I said the same thing in the last two editions).

Immune-based therapy

Treatment for HIV infection designed to affect the immune system and its response to the virus, as opposed to standard antiretroviral therapy, which suppresses the virus itself.

Latency

The ability of HIV to persist in human cells for the lifetime of an infected individual by inserting its DNA into long-lived reservoir cells.

Immune-based therapy is treatment designed to restore the immune system or to improve its ability to fight HIV infection.

Therapeutic vaccine

A vaccine given to treat an existing infection by stimulating the immune system to fight it.

STAYING ON THERAPY

PART EIGHT

Side Effects and Toxicity

What are the side effects of protease inhibitors?

What can I do about changes in my body shape?

How can I protect my liver?

More...

43. What are the side effects of protease inhibitors?

Some side effects and long-term toxicities have been attributed to PIs as a class. These include **gastrointestinal** symptoms, such as loose stools or nausea (Question 66), body shape changes (fat accumulation) (Question 46), and metabolic toxicities, such as increased levels of **cholesterol** and **triglycerides** and high blood sugar or **diabetes**. However, PIs we use today, atazanavir (*Reyataz, Evotaz*) and darunavir (*Prezista, Prezcobix*), are very well tolerated and are much less likely to cause these problems than the older PIs. I suppose I could stop there, but then it would be a short answer, and some of you may still be on the older PIs.

Hyperlipidemia is an elevation of the cholesterol and/or triglyceride levels. High cholesterol can increase the risk for heart disease and stroke (Question 47). Very high triglyceride levels can cause pancreatitis. If you have high lipids on an older drug such as lopinavir/ritonavir (*Kaletra*), consider changing to something more contemporary. You can also modify your diet, perhaps with the help of a nutritionist, and do more aerobic exercise. Depending on how bad the results are and the number of other cardiac risk factors you have, hyperlipidemia may need to be treated either with medications that lower cholesterol and/or triglycerides. The number we worry most about is the LDL ("bad") cholesterol, which we lower with statins (Question 47). Statins are being studied not only for their cholesterol-lowering effects, but also for ability to reduce inflammation, a chronic effect of HIV infection. We're not there yet, but it wouldn't surprise me if someday *everyone* with HIV was on a statin... or maybe just *everyone*.

Insulin resistance means the body can't respond appropriately to the insulin that is produced by the **pancreas** to control blood sugar. When it's severe enough, it can lead to diabetes. We used to think of this as a PI side effect back when we were using indinavir (*Crixivan*), which no one living in the 21st century should still be taking. Insulin resistance is detected with a fasting blood sugar, hemoglobin A1C, or a glucose tolerance test. People with insulin resistance or frank diabetes need to change their diet by avoiding sugars, limiting starches, and eating small amounts throughout the day. Aerobic exercise and weight loss help a lot, but medications are often necessary too.

Fat accumulation (or **lipohypertrophy**) is the buildup of fat in places where it doesn't belong; it is discussed further in Question 46.

Liver toxicity (**hepatotoxicity**) can occur with any PI, but people who have chronic hepatitis B or C are at greatest risk (Question 48). Liver toxicity generally shows up in your blood test results before you feel it yourself. Tell your provider if you develop belly pain, continued nausea, dark urine, or yellow skin or eyes.

Other PI side effects include elevation of **bilirubin** (indinavir, atazanavir), which is completely harmless but may cause jaundice (yellowing of the eyes or skin); kidney stones or kidney damage (indinavir, atazanavir); gallstones (atazanavir); dry skin, hair loss, cracked lips, and ingrown toenails (indinavir); and rash (fosamprenavir or darunavir).

Insulin resistance

A condition in which the body cannot respond to insulin as well as it should. This applies both to insulin naturally produced by the pancreas and insulin injected as medication. Can lead to high blood sugar or diabetes.

Pancreas

An organ in the abdomen that makes insulin and enzymes that help digest food.

Fat accumulation (or lipohypertrophy)

A component of the "lipodystrophy syndrome" in which fat accumulates in abnormal parts of the body, such as inside the abdomen, around the neck, in the breasts, or on the upper back at the base of the neck ("buffalo hump").

Liver toxicity (hepatotoxicity)

Damage to the liver caused by medications.

SIDE EFFECTS AND TOXICITY

Bilirubin

A pigment produced in the liver. When bilirubin levels get too high, the skin and eyes can turn yellow ("jaundice" or "icterus"). Elevated bilirubin can be caused by hepatitis or by two antiretroviral drugs: indinavir (*Crixivan*) or atazanavir (*Reyataz*).

Rose's comment:

The side effects of the protease inhibitors for me are worse during my menstrual cycle. I get diarrhea, abdominal cramps, muscle and joint aches, and gas pain. I know it's the protease inhibitor because I didn't take it for 2 days and the side effects went away. (Joel wasn't happy with me for stopping my meds!!)

Back when I was using drugs like AZT and d4T, my legs got skinny, and I gained weight in my belly. Weight gain is still a problem, though Joel tells me I can't blame it all on the drugs. He claims I should diet and exercise, but what does he know?

Over the years, I've had plenty of other side effects that aren't worth mentioning because they happened with old drugs, and things are a lot better now. But not taking them has never been a question. The side effects have been a small price to pay for my life!

44. What are the side effects of non-nucleoside reverse transcriptase inhibitors (NNRTIs)?

NNRTIs have little long-term toxicity, but they do have short-term side effects you should know about:

- *Rash.* All the NNRTIs can cause a rash, usually during the first few weeks of therapy. It's an itchy, red rash, which often gets better on its own even if you continue the drug. However, severe, even life-threatening rashes can occur, especially with nevirapine (*Viramune*). Signs of a serious rash are peeling or blistering of the skin, sores in the mouth, or fever. Nevirapine is given once a day for the first 2 weeks, then twice a day, but never increase the dose if you have a rash. Rash can occur with efavirenz (*Sustiva, Atripla*), but it's less likely to be severe or to require stopping the drug. Rilpivirine (*Edurant, Complera*) is less likely to cause rash, including severe rash, than either nevirapine or efavirenz.

- *Liver toxicity.* Nevirapine can cause serious, acute liver toxicity during the first few weeks of therapy, especially in women who start the drug with CD4 counts above 250 or men with counts over 400. Always see your provider and get blood tested before you increase the dose of nevirapine after the first 2 weeks. People with chronic hepatitis B or C can take nevirapine, but they are at higher risk for chronic liver toxicity and should be monitored carefully.

- *Hyperlipidemia.* NNRTIs can elevate cholesterol and/or triglycerides. Efavirenz has a greater effect than the other NNRTIs, and now that we're using more "lipid friendly" PIs, efavirenz has become the drug most likely to increase lipids.

- *Neurologic side effects.* Efavirenz often causes vivid dreams (good or bad), dizziness, and concentration difficulties during the first few days or weeks of treatment. Tips on managing these side effects are discussed in Question 52.

45. What should I know about nucleoside analog side effects?

First let's talk about the side effects of drugs from the past that you shouldn't have to know anything about:

- *Peripheral neuropathy.* Stavudine (d4T, *Zerit*) and didanosine (ddI, *Videx*) should no longer be used. They often caused **neuropathy**, that is, damage to the nerves in your feet and legs. The first

Neuropathy (or peripheral neuropathy)

Damage to the nerves resulting in numbness or burning pain, usually in the feet or legs. Can be caused by HIV, some antiretroviral drugs, or other conditions.

symptoms were tingling, numbness, or burning pain in the toes. With time, it could extend up into the legs and become disabling.

Lactic acidosis

A dangerous build-up of lactic acid (lactate) in the blood, which can be caused by some antiretroviral drugs and also by other medical conditions.

Hepatic steatosis ("fatty liver")

A buildup of fat in the liver that can be caused by a variety of medical conditions. When caused by antiretroviral agents, it is often accompanied by lactic acidosis.

- *Lactic acidosis and hepatic steatosis.* **Lactic acidosis** and **hepatic steatosis** are uncommon but serious side effects, mainly of stavudine, but to a lesser degree of zidovudine (AZT, *Retrovir, Combivir, Trizivir*) and didanosine. Symptoms can include shortness of breath, nausea, muscle aches, and just feeling lousy. Of course, these are common symptoms, while lactic acidosis isn't common at all. If you're having them, you may not have lactic acidosis, but you should still report them to your provider. Early diagnosis and an immediate change in therapy are essential, because lactic acidosis can be fatal. You may see lactic acidosis listed as a side effect of the recommended NRTIs (e.g., abacavir, tenofovir), but that's just because they're in the same class as the drugs that *really* cause it.

- *Lipoatrophy.* Fat loss in the face, arms, legs, and buttocks (Question 46) can be caused by stavudine and to a lesser degree by zidovudine and possibly didanosine.

- *Anemia.* Zidovudine can cause anemia. Symptoms include fatigue, dizziness, and shortness of breath. A standard blood test (CBC) will detect anemia.

- *Gastrointestinal side effects.* Zidovudine can cause nausea; tenofovir (TDF, *Viread, Atripla, Complera, Stribild)* can cause nausea, gas, or bloating. NRTIs generally don't cause diarrhea. Didanosine can cause pancreatitis, a dangerous inflammation of the pancreas, and non-cirrhotic portal hypertension, an often fatal liver condition that can occur years after the drug has been stopped.

- *Metabolic toxicity.* Lipid elevation and insulin resistance usually got blamed on PIs, but NRTIs can cause them, too, especially stavudine and zidovudine.

Now on to some toxicities that you really *should* know about:

- *Hypersensitivity.* People taking abacavir (*Ziagen, Epzicom, Trizivir, Kivexa, Triumeq*) can develop a hypersensitivity reaction (HSR) within the first few weeks. HSR feels like the flu and gets worse with each dose. Once you stop abacavir because of possible HSR, you can never take it again; there have been deaths in people who were "re-challenged" with the drug after having had HSR. Fortunately, the risk of HSR has been virtually eliminated by pre-testing for HLA B*5701. If the test is positive, consider yourself allergic and don't take abacavir in any of its forms. If you're negative, you should spend no time worrying about HSR.

- *Kidney toxicity.* Tenofovir can affect the kidneys. The risk is higher if you have kidney problems to begin with, are taking other drugs that affect kidneys, or if you're taking a protease inhibitor. Kidney toxicity is generally gradual and is easily detected by standard blood and urine tests. (Question 49)

- *Loss of bone density.* Starting almost any ART regimen will cause an early loss in bone density. It's generally a small loss and doesn't continue to get worse over time. Tenofovir has more of an effect on bones than other drugs. This is unlikely to be an issue unless you're older or already have poor bone density (Question 50). It's also unlikely to be a problem with tenofovir alafenamide (TAF), a newer version of tenofovir that may be approved by the time you read this (Question 30).

46. *What can I do about changes in my body shape?*

Lipodystrophy

A general term for changes in body shape and fat distribution caused by some antiretroviral agents. Can include lipoatrophy, fat accumulation, or both.

Lipodystrophy is a term used to describe body shape changes that used to occur with older antiretroviral agents. Lipodystrophy includes **lipoatrophy** (fat loss) and fat accumulation. You can have one or the other, or—bad luck!— you can have both. Fortunately, this isn't happening with the drugs we use today, but many people still suffer from the effects of the older drugs they took in the past.

Lipoatrophy

Lipoatrophy

Loss of subcutaneous fat (fat under the skin) in the legs, arms, buttocks, and face, caused by some nucleoside analog reverse transcriptase inhibitors (NRTIs).

Loss of fat in the arms, legs, and buttocks makes your veins stand out and gives you a flat or saggy butt. Loss of fat in the face gives you sunken cheeks and makes you look older or sicker than you are. Stavudine (d4T, *Zerit*) and zidovudine (AZT, *Retrovir, Combivir, Trizivir*) were the most common causes of lipotrophy, but didanosine (ddI, *Videx*) probably caused it too. The best way to deal with lipoatrophy is to avoid the drugs that cause it. If you wait until you've got lipoatrophy and then switch, some fat may return, but it can take a long time and may never return to normal. There are cosmetic procedures that treat lipoatrophy in the face, such as the use of "face filler" injections like polylactic acid (*Sculptra*).

Fat Accumulation

Subcutaneous fat

Fat found under the skin.

Visceral fat

Fat present inside the abdomen, around the internal organs, rather than under the skin.

We used to see fat appear in unusual places, such as the upper back ("buffalo hump"), around the neck, in the breast tissue, or inside the abdomen. As a general rule, belly fat that you can grab between your fingers is **subcutaneous fat** (fat under the skin), which is normal and can't be blamed on your drugs. Abnormal fat is **visceral fat** (fat inside the belly), which can give you a distended, "pregnant-looking" stomach, with fat deep inside that can't be pinched.

The cause of fat accumulation is not completely clear. It was linked to PIs, possibly because of their tendency to increase triglycerides and cause insulin resistance (Question 43). Today, fat gain isn't a side effect of medications at all, but simply the result of improved overall health due to ART. To put it simply, now that you're feeding yourself instead of the virus, you're "catching up"—gaining the weight you *would* have had if you were HIV-negative.

No one should be developing abnormal fat accumulation today, so if you're gaining weight, get off the couch, replace the potato chips with carrot sticks, and get to the gym. Diet and exercise will help, whether you've got abnormal fat accumulation or you're just plain fat. For true visceral fat accumulation, there are treatments that can help, including growth hormone (*Serostim*) and tesamoralin (*Egrifta*), but they are expensive, and the fat tends to return after you stop taking them.

Mike's comment:

I complained to Dr. Gallant about my belly for a couple years. Each time, he'd ask me about my diet and exercise routine. I'd tell him that I couldn't change either. Anyway, I'd decided that the fat was visceral (the kind you can't grab), caused by meds, and that it was my fate to be fat. A couple months ago, my boyfriend decided to lose weight, and I joined him, partly so I wouldn't be rubbing my hollandaise into his face. Lo and behold, eating fewer calories and spending extra time at the gym every day adds up to a lower number on the bathroom scale. I don't know that I'll ever achieve the flat, tomboy stomach of my dreams (what's your opinion, Dr. Gallant?), but working toward a goal seems more productive than sitting on the sofa with a tub of Rocky Road, grousing.

47. Am I at higher risk for heart disease?

Early studies showed that HIV-positive people are at higher risk for heart disease and heart attack than the general population. However, the increased risk was mostly due to the effects of HIV itself, and it is dramatically reduced with ART. Some antiretroviral drugs can increase the risk of heart disease, but they're mostly older drugs that we don't use anymore (Questions 43, 45, and 46). There is an ongoing controversy about whether abacavir (*Ziagen, Epzicom, Trizivir, Triumeq*) increases the risk of heart attack, but I don't usually take that into consideration unless I have a patient who is already at high risk because of many "traditional" risk factors: smoking, diabetes, high blood pressure, high cholesterol, a strong family history of heart disease, or living like a slug.

It's important to put the increased risk in context. First, your risk of a heart attack if you take ART is tiny in comparison to your risk of dying of AIDS if you don't. Second, the risk from even the older, more toxic drugs is still small in comparison to the effects of other risk factors that you have some control over, such as high cholesterol, insulin resistance and diabetes, high blood pressure, smoking, obesity, and physical inactivity. Finally, you lower your cardiac risk by treating HIV far more than you increase it by taking *any* antiretroviral drug.

Here's how to protect your heart: (1) don't smoke, (2) quit smoking, (3) *don't even think about* lighting up that cigarette, (4) get your blood pressure under control if it's high, (5) get your LDL cholesterol down if it's high, (6) keep your blood sugar in control if you've got diabetes, and (7) keep your weight down with aerobic exercise and a healthy diet. That leaves only three other risk factors—getting older, being a man (if you are one), and bad genes—and you can't do anything about them.

... Oh, did I mention that you shouldn't smoke?

48. How can I protect my liver?

The liver is a vitally important organ, though many people are unclear about what it actually does. Its functions are too numerous to list completely, but it's involved in metabolism, the chemical reactions that take place in the cells of the body, including the **detoxification** of many of the drugs we use to treat HIV. It makes proteins, stores fuel for the body, and secretes important hormones and bile, which helps with digestion of food. Because it's so important, I recommend keeping it healthy.

Detoxification

The removal of toxic substances from the body. An important function of the liver and kidneys.

Many antiretroviral drugs can hurt the liver. Almost all of the PIs can cause damage, but usually only in people who have chronic hepatitis B or C. Nevirapine (*Viramune*) can be harmful to the liver, especially in women who start ART with high CD4 counts. Stavudine (d4T, *Zerit*) and zidovudine (AZT, *Retrovir*, *Combivir*, *Trizivir*) can be harmful, too, especially if you also have lactic acidosis. Other medications commonly taken by HIV-positive people, such as cholesterol-lowering drugs, can also cause liver toxicity. Here are some tips for lowering your risk:

1. Get checked for hepatitis A, B, and C. If you're not already immune to A and B, get vaccinated (preferably *after* you've started ART). If you have chronic hepatitis B or C, get evaluated by an expert to start treatment (Questions 79 and

80). In many cases, your HIV provider will also be a hepatitis expert. PCR tests are sometimes necessary to rule out hepatitis, because it's possible to have hepatitis with negative tests.

Transaminases (liver enzymes)

Blood tests used to look for damage to the liver.

2. Get your **transaminases** (**liver enzymes**) checked frequently, especially when you've just started therapy. This is especially important with nevirapine (Question 44).

3. Avoid excessive alcohol use (Question 92). Don't drink at all if you have chronic hepatitis B or C.

4. Use acetaminophen, the active ingredient in *Tylenol* and many other over-the-counter remedies, in moderation; don't use it at all if you have chronic hepatitis.

5. If you're taking medications for hepatitis B, don't stop them. Stopping treatment can cause dangerous hepatitis flares.

Many people use herbal therapies, especially milk thistle, to "detoxify" or protect the liver, though it's not clear whether there's any benefit. Some "natural products" may actually hurt the liver and worsen liver disease. There's no clear evidence that there's anything you can take to protect the liver.

49. Should I worry about my kidneys?

The kidneys are organs that filter your blood and get rid of some of the things you don't need.

The kidneys are organs that filter your blood and get rid of some of the things you don't need. There are only a few things you need to know about the kidneys from an HIV standpoint.

• **HIV-associated nephropathy (HIVAN)**. Black people get the raw end of the deal when it comes to kidney problems. They're at greater risk for kidney failure due to diabetes, hypertension, and also HIV infection. Among HIV-positive blacks, HIVAN is a common cause of kidney failure requiring dialysis or transplantation. The first clue is that there's protein in the urine. The diagnosis is usually made by removing a small piece of the kidney with a needle (**kidney biopsy**). If you've got HIVAN, you should start ART immediately, because it's the only truly effective treatment.

- *Drug toxicity.* Indinavir (*Crixivan*), now rarely used, caused kidney stones and could damage kidney function, which is one of the many reasons we don't use it much anymore. Atazanavir (*Reyataz, Evotaz*) can do the same things, though it's far safer than indinavir. Tenofovir (*Viread, Atripla, Complera, Truvada, Stribild*) can also hurt the kidneys, most often in people who already have kidney problems. If your kidneys aren't working well, then tenofovir may not be the best drug for you, but a newer version, tenofovir alafenamide (TAF), appears to be safer and is expected to be approved soon (Question 30).

- Be careful with other drugs that hurt the kidneys, such as **non-steroidal anti-inflammatory drugs (NSAIDs)** (ibuprofen, naproxen, and related drugs, which are found in many over-the-counter medications, such as *Motrin* and *Aleve*). Most NRTIs should be given at reduced doses if you have kidney problems, even though they don't directly affect the kidneys themselves. HIV-positive people often take other drugs that can cause kidney problems, including **trimethoprim-sulfamethoxazole (TMP-SMX, cotrimoxazole, *Bactrim, Septra*)**.

Kidney problems are detected with standard monitoring tests—the serum creatinine included in the comprehensive chemistry panel and a urinalysis.

Nephropathy, HIV-associated (HIVAN)

A disease of the kidneys caused by HIV infection. It is seen primarily in black patients.

Kidney biopsy

A procedure in which a piece of a kidney is removed using a needle inserted through the skin in order to find out the cause of kidney disorders.

Non-steroidal anti-inflammatory drugs (NSAIDs)

Drugs that are commonly used to suppress inflammation and treat pain. Some are available without a prescription.

Trimethoprim-sulfamethoxazole (TMP-SMX, cotrimoxazole, *Bactrim, Septra*)

An antibiotic used to treat or prevent PCP and to prevent toxoplasmosis.

SIDE EFFECTS AND TOXICITY

50. Are there risks to my bones and joints?

Bone and joint problems can be a complication of HIV infection, HIV therapy, or both. There are two distinct problems—osteopenia/osteoporosis and osteonecrosis:

Osteopenia

A loss of bone density ("thinning of the bones").

Osteoporosis

Severe osteopenia, which can lead to bone fractures.

- **Osteopenia** is loss of bone density. When it becomes severe enough, it's called **osteoporosis** (severe thinning of the bones leading to fractures). You lose some bone density after you start ART, and a little more when the regimen contains tenofovir (*Viread, Truvada, Atripla, Complera, Stribild*), but the amount is small, and bone density generally levels off quickly without progressing further. However, HIV infection probably causes bone loss too, and there's evidence that people who have ever had low CD4 counts are at greater risk for bone fractures. Other risk factors for osteopenia include smoking, use of corticosteroids (prednisone), low testosterone levels (hypogonadism, Question 51), older age, and lower CD4 count. Vitamin D deficiency, a common condition in people with HIV and in the general population, is another risk factor for loss of bone density and may be more common or more severe in people taking efavirenz (*Sustiva, Atripla*). The diagnosis of osteopenia or osteoporosis is made by DEXA scan, which is now recommended as a routine test in HIV-positive men over 50 and post-menopausal women. Taking vitamin D supplements, getting adequate calcium in the diet, and resistance exercise (muscle-building) can also help preserve bone density. ART probably helps, too. Switching from tenofovir to another agent has been shown to increase bone density, and the same will probably be true when we are able to switch people from the current version of tenofovir to the new version, tenofovir alafenamide (TAF, Question 30).

- **Osteonecrosis** is the underlying cause of **avascular necrosis,** a destruction of large joints, usually the hips. We don't know what causes it; we only know it's more common in HIV-positive people. The first symptom is hip pain. Standard x-rays may not detect it; you usually need an MRI of the hips to make the diagnosis. The only treatment is surgical—usually hip replacement.

Osteonecrosis

Damage to bones at the large joints.

Avascular necrosis

Painful joint damage caused by osteonecrosis, usually affecting the hips but sometimes the shoulders.

51. Can HIV or ART affect my hormones?

They can. Here are some examples:

- *Hypogonadism.* HIV-positive men sometimes have low **testosterone** levels (hypogonadism); we see it in men with advanced HIV disease, where it's assumed to be a result of being sick, but also in healthy men on effective ART, where it *may* be a side effect of medications. Symptoms include fatigue, loss of sex drive or performance, weight loss, muscle wasting, or the inability to gain weight. The diagnosis is made with a blood-free testosterone level, which should be drawn in the morning. The condition is treated with testosterone gels, patches, or injections. Gels and patches are preferred because they give you steadier levels and are less likely to shut off your body's own production of testosterone. On that note, let me point out that testosterone should *only* be used in men with low testosterone levels. If your levels are normal, taking testosterone will make your testicles shut down. They'll see no reason to keep producing

Hypogonadism

A deficiency of testosterone, the male sex hormone.

Testosterone

The male sex hormone, which can be low in some HIV-positive men.

SIDE EFFECTS AND TOXICITY

107

*Testosterone
should only
be used in
men with low
testosterone
levels.*

Adrenal insufficiency

A deficiency in the amount of cortisol produced by the adrenal gland.

Cortisol

The steroid hormone produced by the adrenal gland essential to many bodily functions, including the response to stress.

Adrenal gland

A gland in the abdomen that produces cortisol, a steroid hormone that is essential to many bodily functions, including the response to stress.

Cushing's syndrome

Excessive cortisol levels either because of overproduction by the adrenal glands or use of steroid medication.

testosterone themselves, and they'll shrivel up into tiny hazelnuts. If you didn't have hypogonadism before, you'll have it now. Also, remember that it's not *normal* for a 70-year-old retiree to have the testosterone levels of an 18-year-old jock…as much fun as that might be. Your goal should be to maintain levels in the lower end of the normal range, especially as you age. Older men who take excessive doses of testosterone may be at greater risk for heart attack and prostate cancer.

- *Insulin resistance and diabetes.* See Question 43.

- *Thyroid disease.* Thyroid problems aren't much more common in HIV-positive people than in anyone else, but if there's any question, it's easy enough to check using a thyroid-stimulating hormone (TSH) test.

- *Adrenal problems.* **Adrenal insufficiency** (low levels of **cortisol**, a hormone produced by the **adrenal glands**) isn't common except in people with advanced HIV disease, who may be fatigued, dizzy when they stand up, or have blood test abnormalities that are typical for this condition. **Cushing's syndrome** (excessive cortisol) and adrenal insufficiency can occur by combining PIs or cobicistat with certain steroid sprays (fluticasone, which is included in *Flonase* and *Advair*) or steroids that are injected into joints to treat pain (Question 34).

52. Can ART affect my nervous system?

The biggest risk to your nervous system is HIV itself. Untreated HIV infection can lead to a number of unpleasant neurologic problems, discussed further in Question 73. To prevent these problems, take ART.

HIV drugs are mostly safe when it comes to the nervous system, but there are two things you should know about—peripheral neuropathy and efavirenz side effects:

1. *Peripheral neuropathy.* Stavudine (d4T, *Zerit*) and didanosine (ddI, *Videx*) can cause pain or numbness in the feet and legs if you have the misfortune to still be taking these drugs (Question 45).

2. *Efavirenz side effects.* People who take efavirenz (*Sustiva*, *Atripla*) often experience *something* abnormal with the first few doses—dizziness, vivid dreams (enjoyable or otherwise), and "brain fog" or difficulty concentrating, especially in the morning. These symptoms tend to get better with each dose and are often gone within a few days. If they last for more than 3 to 4 weeks, they probably won't get better, and you may need to change medications. Efavirenz is not as widely used in the United States as it once was, but it's still the gold standard in much of the world. If you're taking efavirenz, here are some tips for getting used to it:

   a. Take it in the evening but at least 2 hours after dinner. Taking it with fatty food can increase drug levels and side effects.

   b. Don't take the first dose the night before you have something important to do. Wait until a weekend or a time when you have a few days off.

   c. If you're dreaming so much that you're not getting a good night's sleep, short-term use of a **benzodiazepine** (a tranquilizer in the *Valium* class) may help suppress the dreams. (Benzos should not be used to treat *chronic insomnia*, however. They're habit-forming, and there are much better ways to treat insomnia these days.)

The biggest risk to your nervous system is HIV itself.

Benzodiazepine

A class of drugs used to treat anxiety and insomnia. Diazepam (*Valium*) and alprazolam (*Xanax*) are well known examples. The drugs can be habit-forming and can interact with some antiretroviral drugs.

    d. If you're too groggy in the morning, try taking it earlier in the evening.

    e. Once the side effects go away, you can take it however and whenever you want, as long as you take it each day.

Rarely, efavirenz causes more severe psychiatric symptoms, such as depression or hallucinations. If you find yourself depressed or hearing voices for the first time in your life after recently starting efavirenz, change drugs *now!* If you were depressed before you started the drug, and now you're more depressed, you probably should have picked something else. Long-term effects can occur, too. If you're just "not yourself" in terms of mood or ability to think or focus, talk to your provider about whether efavirenz could be the cause. Sometimes the only way to find out is to switch to a different drug and see what happens.

PART NINE

Opportunistic Infections and Other Complications

What are opportunistic infections?

How do I prevent or treat tuberculosis?

Can HIV cause cancer?

More...

53. What are opportunistic infections?

An "opportunist" is a person who takes advantage of opportunities, usually at the expense of others, for his own benefit. Similarly, an opportunistic infection (OI) is one in which a **pathogen** (a bacterium, virus, fungus, or parasite) takes advantage of a weakness in the body's defense mechanisms to cause disease. In the case of HIV infection, an OI is an infection caused by an organism that is normally kept in check by the **cellular immune system** (the part of the immune system that is most damaged by the HIV virus*).

Some pathogens are exclusively opportunistic, meaning they rarely cause problems in people with normal immune systems. Examples include many of the common HIV-related OIs, such as *Pneumocystis* (Question 54), *Cryptococcus* (Question 57), *Mycobacterium avium* **complex (MAC)** (Question 55), and *Toxoplasma* (Question 56). Other pathogens take advantage of immunosuppressed patients but can cause disease in anyone. Examples are **herpes simplex virus (HSV)** (Question 89), human papilloma virus (HPV), and the bacterium that causes tuberculosis (TB) (Question 59), each of which causes more frequent or severe disease in people with low CD4 counts. As a general rule, "exclusive opportunists" cause disease in people with lower CD4 counts than "optional opportunists."

An OI is an infection caused by an organism that is normally kept in check by the cellular immune system.

In some cases, OIs can be prevented by avoiding exposure to the pathogen itself. For example, we lower the risk of spreading TB by isolating those who are actively infected; you can avoid toxoplasmosis by cooking meat properly; you can avoid syphilis by wearing condoms. However, many opportunistic pathogens are

---

*As opposed to the humoral immune system, which fights infections using antibodies.

"ubiquitous"—they're found everywhere and can't be avoided. Examples include *Pneumocystis*, MAC, and *Cryptococcus*. Prevention of infections caused by these organisms requires either prophylaxis (medical treatment that prevents disease) or better yet, ART, which keeps the CD4 count above the danger zone.

Table 5 lists most of the complications of HIV infection and the CD4 counts at which they occur.

Mike's comment:

After I was diagnosed, I assumed that anything and everything was a symptom of HIV. A cough? It's PCP. Tired after a sleepless night? HIV fatigue. I self-diagnosed thrush and examined my lymph nodes daily (not that I knew where they were or what they were supposed to feel like). If I stumbled, it was a sure sign of nerve trouble. Looking up into the daytime sky to follow the "floaters" was a daily test to self-diagnose CMV retinitis. I wasted many a beautiful summer afternoon that way. I can look back at those days now and smile, if not laugh.

54. What is PCP?

PCP used to stand for *Pneumocystis carinii* pneumonia, one of the most common OIs in HIV-positive patients. *Pneumocystis* started out as a parasite, but microbiologists with way too much time on their hands later decided it was a fungus and changed the name to *Pneumocystis jiroveci*. Knowing there would be a worldwide revolt if they changed the abbreviation to PJP, they kept the PCP abbreviation, which now stands for *Pneumocystis* pneumonia. Clever! Unfortunately, not everyone got the memo, so I often hear younger providers now referring to it as PJP, which makes me old and a little feel queasy.

Mycobacterium avium complex (MAC)

A bacterium related to tuberculosis that causes disease in people with advanced HIV disease, including fever, night sweats, weight loss, diarrhea, liver disease, abdominal pain, and anemia. Also known as *Mycobacterium avium intracellulare* (MAI).

Herpes simplex virus (HSV)

A virus that causes painful blisters and ulcers on the lips, genitals, near the anus, or on other parts of the skin.

PCP

Used to stand for *Pneumocystis carinii* pneumonia, one of the most common OIs in an HIV-positive patient. It now stands for *Pneumocystis* pneumonia, because of the change in the species name.

TABLE 5 Complications of HIV Infection Based on CD4 Count

CD4 count*	Infectious Complications	Noninfectious Complications
Above 500	Acute retroviral syndrome [11, 16]† Vaginal candidiasis [75]	Persistent generalized lymphadenopathy (PGL) [11] Guillain-Barré syndrome [16] Myopathy [16] Aseptic meningitis [16]
200–500	Bacterial pneumonia [67] Pulmonary tuberculosis [59] Shingles (herpes zoster) [71] Oral candidiasis (thrush) [64] Cryptosporidiosis, acute [66, 90] Kaposi's sarcoma [61] Oral hairy leukoplakia (OHL) [64] Cervical and anal dysplasia or cancer [61, 75]	Lymphoma [61] Anemia [70] Thrombocytopenia (low platelet count) [6]
Less than 200	Pneumocystis pneumonia [54] Histoplasmosis [57] Coccidioidomycosis [57] Tuberculosis outside the lungs [59] Progressive multifocal leukoencephalopathy (PML) [73]	Weight loss and wasting [69] Peripheral neuropathy [73] HIV-associated dementia [73]
Less than 100	Toxoplasmosis [56] Cryptococcal meningitis [57] Cryptosporidiosis, chronic [66, 90] Microsporidiosis [66] Candidal esophagitis [65]	
Less than 50	CMV disease [58] MAC infection [55]	Primary central nervous system lymphoma (PCNSL) [61]

* The conditions listed can occur at CD4 counts at or below the ranges shown in this table. Most become more frequent at lower CD4 counts. While uncommon, they can also occur at CD4 counts higher than the ranges listed.

† Numbers in brackets refer to question numbers in this book.

Source: Adapted with permission from Bartlett, JG, Gallant JE, Pham PA. *2012 Medical Management of HIV Infection, 16th ed.* Durham, NC: Knowledge Source Solutions; 2012.

You can't avoid being exposed to *Pneumocystis*. In fact, it may live harmlessly in our lungs already, causing problems only if we become immunosuppressed. You're unlikely to get PCP if your CD4 count is above 200.

The most common symptoms of PCP are gradually worsening shortness of breath, fever, and dry cough. Chest pain and yucky sputum are more typical of bacterial pneumonia, which tends to come on more suddenly.

PCP can be fatal if untreated—it was a common cause of death before we had effective treatment for HIV infection. Clues to the diagnosis include an abnormal chest x-ray and low oxygen levels in the blood. The diagnosis is made by an **induced sputum** exam, which involves inhaling a salt solution that makes you cough hard and deep, or **bronchoscopy**, where a flexible scope is used to sample fluid from your lungs. It's best to confirm the diagnosis rather than just treating it based on the assumption that it's PCP, because other conditions can look just like PCP, the steroids we use to treat PCP can make other OIs worse, and side effects are common during the 3-week course of therapy.

The best treatment for PCP is trimethoprim-sulfamethoxazole (TMP-SMX, cotrimoxazole, *Bactrim*, *Septra*). There are alternatives for people who are allergic to sulfa drugs. People with moderate or severe PCP should also take prednisone, a steroid that keeps your breathing from getting worse before it gets better.

The best way to prevent PCP is to keep your CD4 count well above 200 with ART. Having an undetectable viral load helps too, regardless of your CD4 count. In fact, in a large study, no one who had an undetectable viral load with a CD4 count between 100 and 200 got PCP, even

Induced sputum

A test used to diagnose PCP or tuberculosis in which patients inhale a saline mist that makes them cough deeply. The sputum specimen is then sent to the lab for analysis. Also called "sputum induction."

Bronchoscopy

A diagnostic procedure in which a flexible tube is inserted into the lungs through the mouth (under sedation) so that samples or biopsies can be taken.

The best way to prevent PCP is to keep your CD4 count well above 200 with ART.

PCP can be fatal if untreated—it was a common cause of death before we had effective treatment for HIV infection.

though they weren't taking prophylaxis. Still, prophylaxis is recommended if your CD4 count is below 200 regardless of viral load. The best drug is low-dose TMP-SMX, but there are alternatives. If your CD4 count rises above 200 for at least 3 months, you no longer need prophylaxis. As with other OIs, PCP is much less common than it used to be thanks to effective ART.

55. What is MAC (MAI)?

MAC stands for *Mycobacterium avium* complex. It's also called MAI, for *Mycobacterium avium intracellulare*. It's a bacterium related to tuberculosis (TB), but unlike TB it rarely causes lung disease in people with HIV. Instead it infects the blood, causing fevers, chills, and night sweats. Given enough time, it can infect the bone marrow (causing anemia and low white blood cell counts), the liver (causing abnormal liver function tests), the wall of the intestines (causing wasting and diarrhea), and the lymph nodes (causing belly pain). In advanced HIV disease, MAC is disseminated, which means it's in the bloodstream and spread throughout the body. To make a diagnosis of disseminated MAC, the organism should be grown in culture from a part of the body that's supposed to be sterile—usually the blood, but you can take cultures from bone marrow, the liver, or other internal organs. MAC that's found in the sputum or the stool doesn't count as disseminated infection as it may just be **colonizing** the intestines or lungs—present, but not causing true disease.

Disseminated MAC requires treatment with either **clarithromycin** or **azithromycin** along with **ethambutol** and sometimes **rifabutin**. Treatment clears the blood and suppresses symptoms, but it's not a cure.

Colonization

The presence in the body of microorganisms (viruses, bacteria, etc.) that are not causing symptoms or disease.

Clarithromycin, azithromycin

Antibiotics that can be used to treat or prevent MAC as well as some bacterial lung infections.

Ethambutol

A drug used to treat MAC and TB in combination with other drugs.

Rifabutin

A drug used to treat or prevent MAC. It is also used as an alternative to rifampin to treat tuberculosis.

MAC will return if the drugs are stopped, but if your CD4 count increases on ART to above 100 for at least 6 months, you can stop treatment.

MAC isn't a concern unless your CD4 count is below 50. Should you get to that point, you should take prophylaxis, either with weekly azithromycin or twice-daily clarithromycin. Stopping prophylaxis is possible if your CD4 count rises above 100 for at least 3 months.

MAC isn't a concern unless your CD4 count is below 50.

Like so many other OIs, you can't avoid exposure to MAC because it's everywhere. Prevention with ART or prophylaxis is the only way to prevent getting sick.

56. What is toxo?

"Toxo" is short for toxoplasmosis, a disease caused by the parasite *Toxoplasma gondii*. You get infected either by eating seriously undercooked meat (usually on purpose) or cat poop (usually by accident). After infection, the parasite lives in your body, walled off by the immune system, and causes no harm as long as your immune system remains healthy. However, if your CD4 count falls below 100, you can get sick. The most common and serious form of toxo is **encephalitis**, in which abscesses form in the brain.

A simple blood test, the **anti-*Toxoplasma* IgG antibody test**, will tell you whether you carry the parasite. A positive test means that at some time in your life you were infected. Perhaps as a child you shared a sandbox with Kitty, or maybe as an adult you developed a taste for carpaccio or steak tartar. If your test is positive, keep your CD4 count well above 100 with ART so your immune system can protect you. If it falls below 100, take

Toxoplasma

A parasite (*Toxoplasma gondii*) that causes brain lesions (encephalitis) in people with HIV infection.

Encephalitis

An infection of the brain.

Anti-*Toxoplasma* IgG antibody test

A blood test used to look for exposure to the *Toxoplasma* parasite.

Cryptococcal meningitis

Meningitis (infection of the spinal fluid and spinal cord lining) caused by the fungus *Cryptococcus*.

Meningitis

An infection or inflammation of the spinal fluid and the lining of the spinal cord.

Cryptococcal antigen

A lab test performed on either blood or spinal fluid used to diagnose cryptococcal meningitis.

Spinal tap (lumbar puncture)

A procedure in which a needle is inserted into the back between the vertebrae to collect a sample of cerebrospinal fluid (CSF) to diagnose meningitis.

Amphotericin B

An intravenous drug used to treat serious fungal infections.

Flucytosine (5-FC)

A drug used to treat fungal infections, usually in combination with amphotericin.

Fluconazole

A drug used to treat fungal infections.

prophylaxis, either with trimethoprim-sulfamethoxazole (TMP-SMX, cotrimoxazole, *Bactrim, Septra*) or with one of the alternatives to prevent encephalitis.

If you have a negative antibody test, avoid infection with the parasite, especially if your CD4 count is low. Don't eat raw or rare meat. Wear gloves in the garden, and wash your hands after digging in the dirt. Get someone else to change the litter box for you or use the appropriate precautions. There's no need to trade Kitty in for Fido if you're careful (Question 94). Studies show no increased risk of toxo in cat owners.

Toxoplasmic encephalitis (also called CNS toxo) starts out with headache and/or neurologic symptoms such as seizures or weakness affecting one side of the body. It's treatable, but only with a combination of several unpleasant medications taken at high doses for at least 6 weeks, followed by lower doses until your CD4 count goes up with ART. Prevention is definitely the way to go.

57. What about cryptococcal meningitis and other fungal infections?

Cryptococcal meningitis is an infection of the spinal fluid and lining of the brain with *Cryptococcus*, a yeast (fungus) that is found in the soil and inhaled into the lungs. Although people infected with *Cryptococcus* can develop pneumonia, skin lesions, or other symptoms, most develop **meningitis**, with gradually worsening headache and fever. Unlike bacterial meningitis, which makes you very sick very fast, crypto comes on more gradually. However, if left untreated, it can lead to blindness, deafness, and death. It's unlikely to occur in people with CD4 counts above 100.

A simple blood test, the serum **cryptococcal antigen** (CRAG), is almost always positive in people with cryptococcal meningitis. If it's positive, you need an immediate **spinal tap** (**lumbar puncture**) to confirm the diagnosis and to help determine the severity. Treatment usually involves at least 2 weeks of **amphotericin B** given by vein, often with **flucytosine** (**5-FC**), followed by a long course of **fluconazole**, given by mouth. In severe cases, frequent spinal taps may be needed to lower the spinal fluid pressure during the first few days of therapy. When people die of crypto, which isn't often, it's either because they waited too long to get treated or because they had high spinal fluid pressure that wasn't treated aggressively enough.

Once you've been diagnosed with cryptococcal meningitis, you need to stay on fluconazole to prevent **relapse** until your CD4 count has increased with ART (above 200 for at least 6 months). Because cryptococcal meningitis is easily treatable, unlikely to cause death if treated promptly, and less common than other OIs, we don't use prophylaxis to prevent it. There's no clear way to prevent initial infection with *Cryptococcus*, because it's such a common organism.

While we're on the subject of serious fungal infections, it's worth mentioning a few more. **Candidiasis** is discussed in Questions 64, 65, and 75. **Histoplasmosis** is caused by *Histoplasma capsulatum*, a fungus that's common in the Ohio and Mississippi River Valleys. **Coccidioidomycosis** (**"valley fever"**) is caused by *Coccidioides immitis*, a fungus found in the valleys and deserts of the Southwestern United States and northern Mexico. Both can cause lung disease in people with normal immune systems, but they can cause more severe, widespread disease, including meningitis, in people with low CD4 counts. You can get

Relapse

The return of an illness or disease, usually in someone with a chronic condition.

Canadidiasis

An infection caused by *Candida*, a common yeast.

Histoplasmosis

A disease caused by *Histoplasma capsulatum*, a fungus found mostly in the Ohio and Mississippi River Valleys, which causes lung infection in people with normal immune systems, and infection of the lungs and other organs in people with low CD4 counts.

Coccidioidomycosis ("valley fever")

A disease cause by *Coccidioides immitis*, a fungus found mostly in the deserts and valleys of the southwestern United States and northern Mexico. It can cause lung disease, meningitis, and infection of other organs.

infected by inhaling contaminated dust, and the fungus can live in your body and wait until your CD4 count is low to cause disease. If you're immunosuppressed and you find yourself driving through Indianapolis or the San Joaquin Valley, hold your breath!

58. What is CMV?

Cytomegalovirus (**CMV**) means "big cell virus," because cells infected with CMV are large. CMV is a type of **herpesvirus**, and like all herpesviruses, you can't get rid of it once you've got it. Because it's common and easily transmitted sexually, most people with HIV infection have already been infected.

CMV is rarely a problem for people with normal immune systems, including HIV-positive people with even moderate CD4 counts. You don't have to worry about CMV if your CD4 count is above 50. The most common complication of CMV is **retinitis**, an infection of the retina (the back of the eye), which can lead to blindness if not treated. See an ophthalmologist regularly and report visual changes to your doctor *immediately* if you have a low CD4 count.

The most common complication of CMV is retinitis, an infection of the retina (the back of the eye), which can lead to blindness if not treated.

CMV can also cause gastrointestinal problems, including painful ulcers in the esophagus (**esophagitis**) (Question 64), or infection of the stomach (**gastritis**), small intestines (**enteritis**) or colon (**colitis**), causing diarrhea and abdominal pain. CMV can also affect the nervous system, causing infection of the brain (encephalitis), the spinal cord (**myelitis**), or the spinal nerves (**radiculitis, radiculopathy**).

A positive **anti-CMV IgG** antibody test means you've got the virus. Most HIV-positive people are positive, and there's not much to do about it other than to keep your CD4 count high. If the test is negative, avoid CMV infection: Practice safe sex, and if you should ever need a transfusion, it should be with CMV-negative blood.

59. How do I prevent or treat tuberculosis?

Anyone can get tuberculosis (TB), but the risk is higher for HIV-positive people, increasing as the CD4 count falls. People with low CD4 counts can get more severe TB, which can spread throughout the body, involving organs other than the lungs. You become infected with *Mycobacterium tuberculosis* (the TB bacterium) through close contact with someone who has active TB and is coughing. Infection doesn't always lead to illness. Your body may be able to control the organism on its own, especially if you have a high CD4 count. But if the CD4 count falls, your immune system may no longer be able to protect you.

Everyone with HIV should be tested for TB infection either with a tuberculin skin test (TST, also known as a PPD) or an interferon-gamma release assay (IGRA) blood test such as *QuantiFERON-TB Gold*. A positive test doesn't mean you have TB, but it may mean you've been exposed to the organism and that it's lying dormant in your body (latent tuberculosis infection, or LTBI). If you have LTBI based on a positive test, if you've been in close contact with someone with active TB, or if there's evidence of old TB on your chest x-ray, we generally use

Retinitis

An infection of the retina (the interior surface of the back of the eye), often caused by CMV, that can lead to blindness if not treated.

Esophagitis

Infection or inflammation of the esophagus.

Gastritis

Infection or inflammation of the stomach.

Enteritis

Infection or inflammation of the small intestines.

Colitis

Infection or inflammation of the colon (large intestine).

Myelitis

Infection or inflammation of the spinal cord.

Anyone can get tuberculosis (TB), but the risk is much higher for HIV-positive people.

Radiculitis (radiculopathy)

Infection or inflammation of the nerves that emerge from the spinal cord.

Anti-CMV IgG

A blood test used to look for infection with CMV.

Isoniazid (INH)

A drug used to treat or prevent tuberculosis.

Directly observed therapy (DOT)

A program in which treatment is given to a patient directly by a healthcare professional, at home or in a clinic, in order to ensure that it's taken. Most common with treatment for tuberculosis but sometimes used for HIV therapy.

Dapsone

A drug used to treat or prevent PCP and to prevent toxoplasmosis.

Aerosolized pentamidine

A drug used to prevent PCP.

Atovaquone

A drug used to treat or prevent PCP.

a 9-month course of **isoniazid (INH)** to kill the bacteria and prevent TB. Shorter, 2-drug regimens are not yet recommended for people with HIV. TB tests are less accurate if you're immunosuppressed, so they should be repeated after your CD4 count has increased on ART.

Symptoms of active TB include prolonged fever, night sweats, weight loss, and cough with yucky or bloody sputum; other symptoms depend on the parts of the body involved. The diagnosis is usually made with sputum tests, though bronchoscopy or biopsies of the affected organs may sometimes be necessary. TB is curable with a 6-month course of therapy involving a combination of drugs. Because it's so contagious, treatment is managed by the health department, using **directly observed therapy (DOT)**.

60. How do I prevent opportunistic infections?

Prophylaxis is a fancy term for prevention. When we talk about prophylaxis, we're referring to the use of a drug to prevent an opportunistic infection (OI). If your viral load is undetectable and your CD4 count is high, you don't need to worry, but if your CD4 count is low, here's what you should do to prevent some OIs:

- *PCP.* Start prophylaxis with trimethoprim-sulfamethoxazole (TMP-SMX, cotrimoxazole, *Bactrim*, *Septra*) when your CD4 count is less than 200. If you can't take TMP-SMX use **dapsone**, **aerosolized pentamidine** or **atovaquone** (*Mepron*) (Question 54).

- *Toxoplasmosis.* Start prophylaxis if you have a positive anti-*Toxoplasma* IgG antibody *and* your CD4 count is less than 100. If you're already taking TMP-SMX, you're covered (but make sure you're taking a double-strength tablet daily). If you can't take TMP-SMX, use a combination of dapsone, **pyrimethamine**, and **leucovorin** (**folinic acid**). If your antibody is negative, avoid exposure (Questions 56 and 94).

- *Mycobacterium avium complex (MAC).* Start prophylaxis if your CD4 count is less than 50. Use azithromycin 1,200 mg per week or clarithromycin 500 mg twice a day (Question 55).

- *Cytomegalovirus (CMV).* Prophylaxis isn't recommended. Most people with HIV infection have already been exposed and are at risk for getting sick only if their CD4 count falls below 50 (Question 58).

- *Fungal infections* (Candida *and cryptococcal meningitis*). Unless you've already had one of these infections, prophylaxis isn't recommended (Question 57).

- *Herpes and shingles.* If you've never had these problems, prevention is not recommended. If you have frequent bouts of herpes (several per year), consider chronic suppression with **acyclovir**, **valacyclovir**, or **famciclovir**. Shingles doesn't usually strike more than once, but when it does, prophylaxis is sometimes necessary (Question 89). Live-virus vaccines to prevent chickenpox (*Varivax*) and shingles (*Zostavax*) are available and can be considered in people with CD4 counts above 200.

OPPORTUNISTIC INFECTIONS AND OTHER COMPLICATIONS

Pyrimethamine

A drug used to treat or prevent PCP or toxoplasmosis.

Leucovorin (folinic acid)

A drug used to prevent bone marrow toxicity due to pyrimethamine.

Acyclovir

A drug used to treat herpes simplex and varicella zoster virus.

Valacyclovir

A drug used to treat herpes simplex and varicella zoster virus.

Famciclovir

A drug used to treat herpes simplex and varicella zoster virus.

61. Can HIV cause cancer?

People with HIV infection are at increased risk for certain cancers, though they're far less common than OIs. The cancers most strongly associated with HIV infection are discussed here:

- **Kaposi's sarcoma** (**KS**) was a huge problem during the early years of the epidemic; fortunately, we see very little of it now. It's caused by a virus, **human herpesvirus-8 (HHV-8)**, also known as **Kaposi's sarcoma–associated herpesvirus** (**KSHV**). For reasons that aren't completely understood, KS occurs mostly in gay and bisexual men. It typically causes raised, purple-colored skin lesions, but it can also affect the mouth, lungs, gastrointestinal tract, and other organs. Mild cases can be treated with topical therapies applied to the skin lesions themselves, but more severe cases need to be treated with cancer chemotherapy. Although it often gets better with HIV therapy, KS can sometimes occur even with high CD4 counts.

- Lymphoma doesn't happen often, but it's a serious problem when it occurs. The most common type is **non-Hodgkin's lymphoma** (**NHL**), but people with HIV infection also have an increased risk of **Hodgkin's disease** and **Burkitt's lymphoma**. Lymphoma can pop up just about anywhere in the body and is diagnosed by taking a piece of abnormal tissue (**biopsy**). It responds well to chemotherapy, but the outcome depends on the CD4 count. Being on effective ART can make a big difference.

- Primary central nervous system lymphoma (PCNSL), a lymphoma of the brain, is the cancer you'd *least* want to have. Fortunately, it almost never happens in people with CD4 counts above 50. It's treated with radiation, but in the bad old

Kaposi's sarcoma (KS)

A tumor caused by a virus that is more common in people with HIV infection, especially gay men. Although it usually affects the skin, KS can also affect other parts of the body, including the gastrointestinal tract and lungs.

Human herpesvirus-8 (HHV-8)

The virus that causes Kaposi's sarcoma, Castleman's syndrome, and some rare lymphomas.

Kaposi's sarcoma–associated herpesvirus (KSHV)

An alternative name for human herpesvirus-8 (HHV-8), which causes Kaposi's sarcoma.

Non-Hodgkin's lymphoma (NHL)

The most common type of lymphoma in people with HIV infection.

Hodgkin's disease

A type of lymphoma that is more common in people with HIV but is less common than non-Hodgkin's lymphoma (NHL).

days, the prognosis was miserable. Things are a little better now—still, this is a dreaded complication of advanced HIV disease, to be avoided by taking ART.

- **Cervical cancer** and **anal cancer** are caused by human papillomavirus (HPV), a sexually transmitted virus that causes dysplasia (abnormal cells), which can eventually turn into cancer if not treated. Women should get regular Pap smears to diagnose dysplasia and prevent cancer. Anal Pap smears are now being done, too, especially in women and gay and bisexual men (Question 81). Everyone under 27 should receive the HPV vaccine to help prevent these cancers (Question 26).

I've discussed the most common HIV-related cancers, but it's possible that HIV-positive people may be at higher risk for some of the more "garden variety" cancers as well. Being on ART probably helps; starting it early may help even more. Make sure you're up to date on standard age-based cancer screening tests (colonoscopy, mammogram, prostate-specific antigen [PSA], etc.).

62. What is immune reconstitution?

Immune reconstitution refers to the repair of the immune system with ART. That's usually a good thing, except when it leads to the **immune reconstitution inflammatory syndrome** (IRIS), in which the body's newly restored ability to fight infections creates problems.

Let's use MAC as an example (Question 55). You don't get MAC unless your immune system is severely damaged, usually with a CD4 count below 50. At that point, your immune system is incapable of fighting off the

Burkitt's lymphoma

A type of lymphoma that is seen more frequently in people with HIV infection but is less common than non-Hodgkin's lymphoma (NHL).

Biopsy

A procedure in which a piece of tissue is removed, either with a needle through the skin, through a scope placed in the lungs or gastrointestinal tract, or by a surgical procedure. The specimen is then examined under the microscope and/or submitted for culture to make a diagnosis.

Cervical cancer and anal cancer are caused by human papillomavirus (HPV), a sexually transmitted virus that causes dysplasia (abnormal cells).

Primary central nervous system lymphoma (PCNSL)

A lymphoma involving the brain, seen only in people with advanced HIV disease.

Cervical cancer

A cancer of the cervix (the mouth of the uterus) caused by HPV.

Anal cancer

A cancer of the anus caused by HPV.

Immune reconstitution inflammatory syndrome (IRIS)

A condition that sometimes occurs in people with low CD4 counts who start ART in which the improved immune system reacts to organisms (such as MAC, the TB bacterium, or fungi), causing illness, including fevers, weight loss, swollen lymph nodes, or abscesses.

Progressive multifocal leukoencephalopathy (PML)

A viral infection of the brain caused by JC virus, which results in progressive neurologic deterioration.

MAC bacteria that are running rampant in the body. However, if you start ART when you have MAC, your immune system may recover enough to start doing its job. It will form walls around the bacteria, leading to abscesses or enlarged, inflamed lymph nodes. The immune response may cause fever, night sweats, and weight loss.

IRIS can occur with a variety of organisms. The most common are MAC and TB, but it can also happen with CMV, *Pneumocystis*, *Cryptococcus,* and others. People sometimes have outbreaks of shingles or herpes after they start ART. Even Kaposi's sarcoma and **progressive multifocal leukoencephalopathy** (**PML**), which usually get better with ART, can sometimes get worse.

As unpleasant as IRIS can be, it's temporary and a sign that your immune system is recovering. In almost all cases, you should continue ART. It's important to find out what the underlying OI is, usually with a biopsy, and then treat it. Steroids (prednisone) are sometimes used to help get people through IRIS by blunting the immune response to the organism while still allowing ART to suppress HIV. The prednisone dose can be gradually lowered until the symptoms are gone.

63. Will HIV or ART make me age faster?

There's been a lot of talk recently about "accelerated aging" with HIV infection. The term is scary and a little misleading. It doesn't mean you'll get gray hair and wrinkles sooner, or that the overall aging process is being sped up, or that you're on a faster pace to the grave. Instead, it refers to the fact that some of the complications of aging are being seen more often or at younger ages in some HIV-positive people. Examples include heart disease, osteoporosis, cancer, and changes in brain function, including dementia.

There are many unanswered questions about HIV and aging, which is now the subject of a great deal of speculation as well as scientific research:

1. *Is "premature aging" caused by HIV, ART, or both?* HIV itself is mostly to blame. People who start ART with low CD4 counts are at greater risk for heart disease, bone fractures, and cognitive impairment (brain disease). People who spend a lot of time with high viral loads are at greater risk of lymphoma and other complications. ART goes a long way toward preventing the long-term complications of HIV, but ART isn't completely off the hook, because treatment with some drugs may increase the risk of kidney disease, loss of bone density, and atherosclerosis. We do know that ART does a lot more good than harm.

2. *How does HIV accelerate aging?* I've talked before about the inflammation and immune activation that occur with HIV infection (Question 9). These are the most likely reasons for the increased risk of aging complications. ART dramatically reduces these processes, which explains many of its long-term benefits.

3. *Can HIV cause premature aging despite effective ART?* ART clearly slows this process, but we don't know whether starting ART early, at a high CD4 count, will completely eliminate the long-term risks. People on ART have much lower levels of inflammation and immune

activation than people who aren't being treated, but their levels may still be slightly higher than in HIV-negative people. We'll need more time to find out whether someone with optimally treated HIV infection can expect the same quality of life as someone without HIV infection.

For now, the best way to stay healthy into your old age is to keep your viral load suppressed on ART, and then follow all the many recommendations we're given to become healthy, vigorous senior citizens.

PART TEN

Symptoms

What can I do about nausea and diarrhea?

What if I get a cold or the flu?

Why am I so tired?

More...

64. What's wrong with my mouth?

The most common cause of mouth and throat problems is **oropharyngeal candidiasis** ("thrush"), a buildup of *Candida* (a common yeast or fungus). Thrush is easy to diagnose with a mirror and a flashlight. You'll see whitish-yellow, curd-like patches, especially on the roof and sides of the mouth, the back of the throat, and the gums. These patches can be easily scraped off. Don't confuse a white coating on the tongue with thrush. The tongue is usually the last part of the mouth to be infected, and a white coating on the tongue, with no other evidence of thrush, is usually just...a white coating on the tongue.

Thrush can also be confused with **oral hairy leukoplakia** (**OHL**), a condition caused by **Epstein-Barr virus** (**EBV**) that looks like a white racing stripe down both sides of the tongue. Unlike thrush, it can't be scraped off. *Candida* can cause other mouth problems besides thrush—**erythematous candidiasis** (redness on the roof of the mouth that is sometimes painful) and **angular cheilitis** (cracks at the corners of the lips).

Painful ulcers in the mouth can be caused by viruses, but they're more often **aphthous ulcers**. "Aphthous" is a good word for a spelling bee that essentially means that we have no idea about the cause. The diagnosis of most of these conditions is usually based on appearance alone; special tests aren't necessary.

Thrush and OHL are fairly benign conditions, but they both indicate that something's seriously wrong with your immune system and that you should have started ART earlier. Thrush is treated with antifungal medication: either oral fluconazole or medications that treat

---

Oropharyngeal candidiasis

Candida (yeast) infections involving the mouth and throat, including thrush, angular cheilitis, and erythematous candidiasis.

Candida

A fungus (yeast) that can cause thrush, esophagitis, and vaginitis in people with HIV infection.

Oral hairy leukoplakia (OHL)

Painless white plaques, or "stripes," on the sides of the tongue caused by Epstein-Barr virus.

Epstein-Barr virus (EBV)

A herpesvirus that causes infectious mononucleosis ("mono"), oral hairy leukoplakia, and some lymphomas.

Thrush and OHL are fairly benign conditions, but they both indicate that something's seriously wrong with your immune system.

---

only the surfaces, such as **clotrimazole troches** (lozenges) or **nystatin** mouth rinses. Because it's harmless, we don't usually treat OHL except with ART.

Before we leave the mouth, don't forget your teeth and gums. People with low CD4 counts are at risk for serious mouth infections. Brushing, flossing, and seeing a dentist and oral hygienist on a regular basis are important to keep your teeth and gums in good shape.

65. Why does it hurt to swallow?

There are two medical terms for swallowing symptoms—**dysphagia** (difficulty swallowing) and **odynophagia** (painful swallowing), but the distinction is less important than the location. Is the problem confined to the back of the throat (**pharynx**) or does it extend into the chest (**esophagus**)? For mouth and throat symptoms, see Question 64.

When the problem is in the chest, it can be a sign of esophagitis, an inflammation of the esophagus, the tube that connects your throat with your stomach. The most common cause is *Candida,* the same yeast (fungus) that causes thrush and **vaginitis**. People with *Candida* esophagitis usually have a CD4 count below 100. Since *Candida* is the most common cause of esophagitis, the usual approach is to treat with fluconazole and see what happens. If *Candida* is the cause, you'll be swallowing easier within a day or two. If not, you'll need an **endoscopy**, an outpatient procedure in which a flexible tube with a camera is passed from the mouth into the esophagus so that pictures and biopsies can be taken.

SYMPTOMS

Erythematous candidiasis

An infection of the mouth caused by *Candida* in which the roof of the mouth (palate) becomes red and sometimes painful.

Angular cheilitis

Cracking of the corners of the lips, sometimes caused by Candida.

Aphthous ulcers

Painful ulcers in the mouth (aphthous stomatitis) or esophagus (aphthous esophagitis) that can occur in people with HIV. The cause is unknown.

Clotrimazole troches

Antifungal lozenges used to treat thrush.

Nystatin

An antifungal mouth rinse used to treat thrush.

Dysphagia

Difficulty swallowing.

Odynophagia

Painful swallowing.

Pharynx

Throat.

Candida is the most common cause of esophagitis.

Esophagus

The tube that connects the mouth and throat to the stomach.

Vaginitis

Infection or inflammation of the vagina.

Endoscopy

A medical procedure in which a flexible tube is inserted into the esophagus and stomach through the mouth, while the patient is sedated, in order to take samples or biopsies or to treat a variety of conditions.

Other causes of esophagitis are herpes simplex virus (HSV), cytomegalovirus (CMV), and aphthous ulcers, each of which causes painful ulcers in the wall of the esophagus. The treatment of these conditions depends on the cause. Drug-resistant *Candida* can also cause esophagitis and must be treated with other antifungal drugs.

Of course, HIV-positive people can also develop the same esophageal problems that HIV-negative people get, including esophageal reflux, spasm, or strictures. Pills can get stuck on the way down and irritate the esophagus, so always take your meds with plenty of water.

66. What can I do about nausea and diarrhea?

In HIV-positive people, nausea can be caused by medications. Zidovudine (AZT, *Retrovir, Combivir, Trizivir*) and some of the older protease inhibitors were the most common offenders. If your nausea began as soon as you started a new drug, then there's no mystery about the cause. In some cases, the nausea may improve with time or by taking the pills with food. Your doctor can also prescribe medications for nausea, but if the problem persists, you may have to change drugs, and that would be the first thing I'd do in someone taking an outdated drug like AZT. If you've developed nausea but haven't recently changed or added medications, then it's important to look further for a cause.

Diarrhea can be caused by medications, too, especially some of the older PIs. The best way to treat drug-related diarrhea—aside from switching drugs—is with daily fiber supplements, such as psyllium. Don't be put off by the word "laxative" on the bottle. Fiber supplements add bulk to the stool, which is a good thing whether you've got diarrhea or constipation. If they don't work, ask your doctor about prescribed or over-the-counter anti-diarrhea medications, or about making a change in your regimen.

There are many infectious causes of diarrhea, including common viruses, bacteria, and parasites. Some of these organisms, such as *Cryptosporidium*, **microsporidia**, *Isospora* (which causes **isosporiasis**), and *Salmonella* are opportunistic—they occur or are more severe because of immunosuppression. Advanced HIV infection itself can also cause diarrhea. If you have prolonged diarrhea that's not caused by medications, you'll need to be evaluated: first with stool studies, and if those are negative, with a scope (flexible tube with a camera), either from above (endoscopy), from below (**colonoscopy**), or both.

Diarrhea caused by viruses or food poisoning usually gets better on its own after a few days, but get medical attention if you have persistent diarrhea, or if you have fever, belly pain, blood in your stool, or dizziness. When you have diarrhea, eat a bland diet with no milk products, and hydrate, hydrate, hydrate!

Mike's comment:

Fiber supplements work. They work for diarrhea caused by PIs, and they work for constipation caused by calcium supplements. Some types are more palatable and work better than others. The one I am using these days is right tasty. I take it with both my morning and evening meds. Neither the capsules nor the chewables work as well for me as the powder that I add to a glass of water. I have found a few brands that I like, and I switch between flavors before I get too sick of any one. When I skip a serving, I can tell the difference, and the change isn't for the better.

SYMPTOMS

Cryptosporidium

The parasite that causes crypto-sporidiosis, which can cause chronic diarrhea in immuno-suppressed people. The organism can be found in contaminated water or transmitted from person to person.

Microsporidia

A variety of opportunistic parasites that cause chronic diarrhea in people with low CD4 counts.

Isosporiasis

A disease caused by the parasite *Isospora belli*, which causes chronic diarrhea in people with low CD4 counts. Uncommon in the United States and other developed countries.

Salmonella

A group of bacteria that can cause severe diarrhea, fever, and bloodstream infections.

Colonoscopy

A medical procedure in which a flexible scope is inserted into the rectum and colon through the anus, while the patient is sedated, in order to look for abnormalities and take biopsies.

67. *What do I do about cough or shortness of breath?*

The possible causes of cough or shortness of breath depend on your CD4 count. If it's well above 200, then the list is essentially the same as it would be in an HIV-negative person. Cough can be due to the common cold, bronchitis, pneumonia, asthma, smoking, the use of certain medications, or esophageal reflux (stomach acid going up into the esophagus instead of staying in the stomach). Shortness of breath can be due to asthma, pneumonia, anemia, or acidosis (a buildup of acid in your blood). The kind of cough you get with a common cold or bronchitis doesn't usually require medical attention (Question 68). If you recently had a cold and now have one of those nagging, hacking coughs that gets worse when you laugh, exercise, or go out in the cold, you may have **bronchospasm** (or **reactive airways**), which can be treated with an inhaled bronchodilator such as albuterol.

The same is true if your CD4 count is low, except that now there's a longer list of possible causes. If your count is below 200, you may have PCP. With a count less than 100, there's a risk for pneumonia caused by *Cryptococcus*, *Toxoplasma*, or *Histoplasma*, which are less common than PCP (Question 54). HIV-positive people are at much higher risk for TB at any CD4 count, and the risk gets higher as the CD4 gets lower (Question 59).

You should get medical attention if you have a severe cough or one that doesn't get better with time, or if you have a high fever, chest pain when you take a deep breath, or are coughing up blood. You should never ignore shortness of breath or any change in your ability to exert yourself. If you're winded after climbing one

Bronchospasm (or reactive airways)

The tendency of the bronchi (airways in the lung) to constrict (narrow), causing shortness of breath or cough. This can be chronic (in patients with asthma, for example) or temporary, following an upper respiratory infection.

You should never ignore shortness of breath or any change in your ability to exert yourself.

flight of stairs but could climb three flights a month ago, you need to get checked out.

68. What if I get a cold or the flu?

HIV-positive people get colds and flu just like everyone else. The symptoms and duration of the illness are the same, and they're at no greater risk from complications. That's because viruses that cause the cold and flu are controlled by the **humoral** (antibody-mediated) **immune system**, not the cellular immune system that uses CD4 cells and is damaged by HIV.

For that reason, you don't need to do anything special if you get a cold—just rest, drink fluids, and take whatever over-the-counter cold remedy will treat the symptoms you're experiencing. These medications don't interact with HIV drugs, and you're unlikely to get anything better by prescription. *You don't need antibiotics!* Your illness is caused by a virus; antibiotics kill only bacteria. They're often prescribed as placebos to keep patients happy and coming back, which is contributing to a huge drug resistance problem worldwide. This applies to **bronchitis** and most forms of **sinusitis** and sore throat as well. Studies have shown that antibiotics are no better than placebo to treat bronchitis. Cough medicine and sometimes an inhaled bronchodilator may help you feel better, but as with the common cold, you just have to ride it out. Sore throats require antibiotics only if they're caused by group A strep (**strep throat**) or gonorrhea, but otherwise they're viral and should be treated with throat lozenges. Most people with colds will have sinus congestion at some point. Sinusitis should only be treated with antibiotics if it's severe or prolonged. When an adult has ear pain during a cold, it's rarely an ear

SYMPTOMS

Humoral immune system

The part of the immune system that uses antibodies to fight infection.

Bronchitis

An infection of the bronchi (airways), usually caused by a viral infection and often occurring after a common cold.

Sinusitis

An infection of the sinuses—air spaces in the head connected to the nasal passages.

Strep throat

The common term for streptococcal pharyngitis, a bacterial infection of the throat caused by group A beta-hemolytic *Streptococcus*.

infection, but usually just congestion of the Eustachian tubes, treated with decongestants. If we want to have antibiotics around to treat serious bacterial infections, we need to stop using them to treat viral infections that get better just as fast on their own.

Pneumonia

An infection of the air spaces of the lungs, which can be caused by a variety of infectious organisms.

The one infection we *do* want to treat with antibiotics is **pneumonia**, which will usually give you some combination of fever, cough, chest pain, and/or shortness of breath. It will feel much worse than the common cold or bronchitis. There is *no* evidence to support the use of antibiotics to prevent a cold from "going into the chest" or "preventing pneumonia." They're completely different diseases.

Get a flu shot every fall. If you develop true influenza during flu season, the use of anti-influenza drugs can shorten the course of the illness a little, but only if used within the first few days.

69. Why am I losing weight?

During the dark days before effective ART, weight loss was almost universal as AIDS progressed, and many patients wasted away to nothing before they died. Weight loss is uncommon now that we have effective therapy for HIV infection, and it's usually caused by something else. Here are some common, treatable causes of weight loss:

1. *Untreated HIV infection.* If you're losing weight because of HIV infection, you need to be on ART. Weight loss is more likely to occur if you have a high viral load.

2. *Hypogonadism.* Men with low testosterone levels can lose weight (Question 51). Check your

thyroid function while you're at it with a TSH (thyroid-stimulating hormone) level.

3. *Depression.* This is a common cause of weight loss, because depressed people often lose their appetites (Questions 82 and 83).

4. *Lipoatrophy.* This doesn't usually cause loss of total body weight, but it can make you look like you've lost weight (Question 46).

5. *Gastrointestinal disorders.* Problems in the esophagus could make it harder to swallow; nausea and vomiting could make you less likely to eat or to absorb your food; you could also have a problem with absorption of nutrients in the small intestine.

In the past, we often used anabolic steroids to help people gain muscle mass as they wasted away from AIDS. It wasn't a solution to the problem, but it helped control the symptoms. I don't see wasting anymore, but I do see men who want to use their HIV status as an excuse to get big muscles without having to spend as much time at the gym. That's *not* a good idea. If I thought anabolic steroids were safe, *I'd* be ripped!

70. Why am I tired?

Fatigue is common among HIV-positive people... and HIV-negative people too, for that matter. I'm fatigued myself, and I've still got 30 more questions to go! If you're experiencing an unusual amount of fatigue, consider the following possible causes:

Fatigue is not something you should have to live with.

• *Depression.* This may be the most common reason for fatigue. People with depression have no energy, but they also have a number of other symptoms, discussed in Question 82.

- *Insomnia* or *sleep apnea.* Not getting enough sleep at night will obviously make you tired and sleepy during the day.

- *Anemia.* In addition to fatigue, people with anemia may be pale, dizzy, and short of breath. Causes include medications, especially zidovudine (AZT, *Retrovir, Combivir, Trizivir*), dietary deficiencies, HIV-related complications, and HIV itself. Anemia is easy to diagnose with a simple blood count, but further tests are then necessary to determine the cause.

Anemia is easy to diagnose with a simple blood count.

- *Hormone deficiencies.* These include low testosterone levels (hypogonadism), thyroid hormone deficiency (**hypothyroidism**), and adrenal insufficiency (Question 51).

Hypothyroidism

A deficiency in thyroid hormone.

- *Medications.* Zidovudine is known to cause fatigue even when it's not causing anemia. Efavirenz (*Sustiva, Atripla*) can do it, too, especially in the first few weeks if it's disturbing your sleep with lots of wild dreams (Question 52).

- *Lactic acidosis.* This is an uncommon but serious side effect of stavudine (d4T, *Zerit*), zidovudine, and possibly didanosine (ddI, *Videx*). Lactic acidosis causes other symptoms as well, which are discussed in Question 45.

- *HIV infection.* Fatigue is common in people with high viral loads and/or low CD4 counts, or when there's significant wasting.

Because virtually all of the causes of fatigue are treatable, it's important to make the diagnosis. Fatigue is not something you should have to live with.

71. Can HIV affect my skin?

Skin problems can be caused by HIV itself, by complications of HIV, and by medications. It's hard to talk about skin problems in a book with no color pictures, and I don't have room to talk about treatment. If you're having skin problems, see your provider or a dermatologist. Here's an incomplete list of things that can go wrong with the skin:

- **Abscesses** ("boils") have become common due to the epidemic of community-acquired **methicillin-resistant** *Staphylococcus aureus* (**MRSA**). They usually have to be opened up and drained. It's important to culture the pus first so that the right antibiotic can be chosen.

- Drug reactions often begin with a red, itchy rash. They can be caused by the NNRTIs, some PIs, especially fosamprenavir (*Lexiva*) and darunavir (*Prezista, Prezcobix*), trimethoprim-sulfamethoxazole, and many other medications.

- **Folliculitis** causes raised, itchy, red bumps in areas where there's hair. It can be caused by bacteria, *Demodex* mites, or can be "eosinophilic," a term used to describe the type of cells that are seen on a biopsy.

- Herpes simplex can affect the lips, the genitals, the area around the anus, or other parts of the skin. It causes small, painful blisters that open up and become shallow ulcers on a red base.

- Kaposi's sarcoma causes raised purple lesions on the skin or in the mouth (Question 61).

- *Molluscum contagiosum* lesions are raised, skin-colored, fleshy bumps with small indentations in the middle. They can occur anywhere but are especially common on the genitals, face, and neck.

- Opportunistic infections can cause skin problems, including cryptococcosis, histoplasmosis, and

Abscesses

Collections of pus (infectious organisms and white blood cells) in the skin ("boil") or other parts of the body.

Methicillin-resistant *Staphylococcus aureus* (MRSA)

A drug-resistant bacterium that traditionally caused serious illness in seriously ill, hospitalized patients but that has recently become a common cause of skin disease, including abscesses (community-acquired MRSA).

Folliculitis

Infection of the hair follicles and skin around them.

Molluscum contagiosum

Flesh-colored bumps or protuberances on the skin that are caused by a poxvirus and can be sexually transmitted.

Bartonella

A bacterium that can cause skin disease (bacillary angiomatosis) or liver disease (peliosis hepatis) in people with HIV.

SYMPTOMS

Bacillary angiomatosis

A bacterial skin disease caused by *Bartonella*, which causes raised purple lesions on the skin sometimes confused with Kaposi's sarcoma.

Prurigo nodularis

A condition characterized by itchy bumps on the skin, seen more commonly in people with HIV.

Psoriasis

A skin condition that results in dry, scaly, itchy plaques on the skin that can get worse with immunosuppression due to HIV infection.

Scabies

An itchy skin condition caused by a mite that burrows under the skin and can be spread to others by close contact.

Seborrheic dermatitis

A common skin condition causing flakiness on the face, especially around the eyebrows and in the folds on the cheeks.

Tension headache

A headache caused by muscle tension.

Bartonella (**bacillary angiomatosis**). A skin biopsy is usually the best way to make the diagnosis.

- **Prurigo nodularis** sounds exotic, but it's just a way to say "itchy bumps" in Latin. This may be a reaction to too much scratching over a long period of time.

- **Psoriasis** can get worse or appear for the first time in people with low CD4 counts. It causes itchy raised patches, especially on the elbows, knees, and buttocks.

- **Scabies** is caused by a common skin mite. It causes intense itching, especially at night. A common location is on the backs of the hands and between the fingers. It can be severe in people with low CD4 counts.

- **Seborrheic dermatitis** causes a flaky, red rash on the face, especially in the folds on the cheeks and around the eyebrows.

- Secondary syphilis can cause a variety of rashes, including red bumps, sometimes involving the palms and soles (Question 89).

- Shingles is reactivation of varicella zoster virus (VZV), the chickenpox virus, in the skin over a single nerve. It causes painful blisters in a confined, band-like area on one side of the body.

72. Why do I have a headache?

If your CD4 count is over 100 and you've got a headache, it's probably due to one of the usual causes—tension headache, migraine, or sinus headache. A **tension headache** feels like a band-like tightness or constriction, tends to come on later in the day, and is present on both sides of the head. A **migraine** can occur at any time of the day, is often present on one side of the head, may be throbbing, and may occur with visual changes or nausea. People with a **sinus headache** have sinus congestion, a feeling of fullness or pressure below the eyes or in the forehead, and sometimes plentiful thick snot.

If your CD4 count is below 100 and you have a headache, especially a chronic headache that gets gradually worse, possibly with fever or stiff neck, you should be checked for cryptococcal meningitis (Question 57). A simple blood test, the serum cryptococcal antigen, will determine whether cryptococcal meningitis is likely. If the test is positive, you need an immediate spinal tap to confirm the diagnosis and to find out the severity. Other types of meningitis (bacterial, *Listeria*) are far less common but come on more suddenly. They can also start out with a headache and fever.

If you also have neurologic changes (seizures, weakness, or numbness on one side of the body; coordination problems; or mental changes), you could have a mass in the brain, usually caused by either toxoplasmosis (Question 56) or a brain lymphoma (Question 61). The first step here is an MRI scan of the brain with contrast injected through the vein. Progressive multifocal leukoencephalopathy (PML), which is caused by **JC virus**, can also cause neurologic symptoms, but it's less likely to cause a headache.

73. Can HIV affect my nervous system?

Untreated HIV infection can wreak havoc your nervous system. The virus gets into the brain and spinal fluid and can lead to a lot of unpleasant complications, some of which are permanent. The way to prevent these

Migraine headache

A severe headache, often on one side of the head, sometimes accompanied by visual changes or nausea.

Sinus headache

A headache caused by congestion of the sinuses.

Listeria

A foodborne bacterium that can cause meningitis and other infections. Although not common, the risk for acquiring Listeria is higher in people with HIV.

If your CD4 count is below 100 and you have a headache, especially a chronic headache that gets gradually worse, possibly with fever or stiff neck, you should be checked for cryptococcal meningitis.

SYMPTOMS

JC virus

The cause of progressive multifocal leukoencephalopathy (PML).

Neuro-psychological testing

A series of tests, usually performed by a psychologist or neurologist, to assess memory and thinking skills. Can be used to diagnose dementia, or to determine whether someone has depression or dementia.

The most common cause of memory loss is depression, which can sometimes look very much like dementia.

problems is to take ART as soon after diagnosis as possible. I'll discuss the approach to some neurologic symptoms here:

- *Headache.* See Question 72.

- *Memory loss or personality changes.* The most common cause of memory loss is depression, which can sometimes look very much like dementia. It's possible to tell the difference with special memory and cognitive tests (**neuropsychological testing**), but if there's any question, a few weeks of treatment with an antidepressant may help sort it out (Questions 82 and 83). If you're experiencing memory loss but aren't depressed, then it's important to find out whether you have HIV dementia or other HIV-related brain complications.

- *Foot or leg pain or numbness.* The most common cause of peripheral neuropathy is toxicity from stavudine (d4T, *Zerit*) or didanosine (ddI, *Videx*). Untreated HIV can cause this too. The treatment is to start taking an ART regimen that doesn't include stavudine or didanosine (Question 45).

- *Seizures.* Anyone who has a seizure for the first time should go to an emergency room. A CT or MRI scan of the brain will be ordered to look for masses or lesions.

- *Weakness, coordination problems, unsteady gait, or incontinence.* Depending on the location of the symptoms, you will need an MRI scan of the brain and/or spinal cord.

PART ELEVEN

Women's Issues, Pregnancy, and Children

How is HIV infection different for women?

What if I want to get pregnant?

What if my child is HIV positive?

More...

74. How is HIV infection different for women?

HIV infection in women is similar to HIV infection in men, but there are a few important differences. HIV-positive women tend to have lower viral loads than HIV-positive men at the same CD4 counts. This shouldn't affect the decision of when to start treatment now that treatment is recommended for everyone.

Some studies suggested that HIV-positive women die sooner than HIV-positive men, but that was because of delayed diagnosis. Women at risk for HIV may have less access to health care. If they were infected hetero-sexually, they may not realize they're at risk and avoid testing. Women who get diagnosed and treated for HIV infection live as long as men—longer, in fact, since women generally tend to outlive men.

Women respond well to ART. There are no HIV drugs that can't be used in women or that are specifically recommended for women, but there are some gender-specific issues to be aware of. Nevirapine (*Viramune*) is more likely to cause liver toxicity in women than in men, and it's not recommended for women starting treatment with CD4 counts above 250. Efavirenz (*Sustiva, Atripla*) can cause birth defects if given during the first trimester of pregnancy, so we generally avoid it in women who are trying to become pregnant or who aren't trying to prevent it (Question 76). A number of PIs and NNRTIs may decrease the effectiveness of birth control pills, making them unreliable. Women taking drugs that interact with birth control pills should use an additional form of contraception, such as condoms or a diaphragm.

75. Does HIV cause gynecologic problems?

A number of common gynecologic problems can be more frequent or severe in HIV-positive women. *Candida* vaginitis (a vaginal infection cause by *Candida,* a common yeast) is a good example. More recurrent or serious candidiasis is sometimes the first sign of immunosuppression in HIV-positive women. Vaginitis can be treated with topical antifungal agents or with oral fluconazole.

Bacterial vaginosis, a bacterial infection that causes vaginal discharge, is also more common in women with HIV. **Pelvic inflammatory disease** (**PID**), an infection of the uterus and fallopian tubes usually caused by sexually transmitted infections, can sometimes be more serious and may be more likely to require surgery in HIV-positive women.

As in men, genital herpes can be more severe or recur more frequently as the CD4 count falls. It causes painful genital ulcers that should be treated with anti-herpes medications. Genital herpes can increase the viral load and can make it easier to transmit HIV. Women who have frequent herpes outbreaks should take daily medication to prevent flares. HIV-positive women can also develop idiopathic genital ulcers—ulcers for which no cause is found. These are similar to aphthous ulcers in the mouth and esophagus (Questions 64 and 65). They usually occur in women with very low CD4 counts and are best treated with ART, along with the advice of a gynecologist who is also an expert in treating HIV-positive women.

Bacterial vaginosis

A bacterial infection of the vagina that causes vaginal discharge.

Pelvic inflammatory disease (PID)

A serious infection of the uterus and fallopian tubes usually caused by sexually transmitted infections, especially gonorrhea and chlamydia.

Women respond well to ART. There are no HIV drugs that can't be used in women or that are specifically recommended for women.

WOMEN'S ISSUES, PREGNANCY, AND CHILDREN

Human papillomavirus (HPV) (Question 81) causes genital warts, cervical dysplasia, and cervical cancer.

Rose's comment:

Before I was diagnosed, I'd been battling yeast infections for 2 years, but the doctors didn't pick up on it. After I was diagnosed, I learned that frequent or severe yeast infections can be a sign of HIV infection in women. I also had abnormal Pap smears caused by the HPV virus. HIV puts me at more risk for cervical problems than other women. Freezing didn't work, and I had to get a cone biopsy where they cut the bad cells out of your cervix, just like coring an apple. It's important for HIV-positive women to get regular pelvic exams and Pap smears.

76. What if I want to get pregnant?

Pregnancy is a completely realistic option for HIV-positive women now that we can treat HIV effectively and prevent infection in the baby. However, pregnancy should be carefully planned and monitored in HIV-positive women.

All pregnant women should be on ART, ideally started before they become pregnant. ART is a *must* after the first trimester, because transmission to the baby is extremely unlikely if Mom's viral load is undetectable at delivery. We have the best safety data in pregnancy on two PIs: lopinavir/ritonavir (*Kaletra*) and atazanavir (*Reyataz*) boosted with ritonavir (*Norvir*). Guidelines recommend that one of these be combined with zidovudine/lamivudine (*Combivir* or generic). I generally use atazanavir, as it's better tolerated than lopinavir/ritonavir, but I prefer to combine it with tenofovir/emtricitabine

(*Truvada*), an acceptable alternative to *Combivir* that has fewer side effects. (Pregnant women suffer from enough nausea already without having to suffer more on AZT!)

Although we advise women not to get pregnant if they're taking efavirenz, it's widely used in young women who live in resource-limited settings. Even in the United States, where we have a lot more malpractice attorneys, there's no reason to switch from efavirenz if you become pregnant, since the window for the birth defect of concern (neural tube defects) has already closed. Nevirapine (*Viramune*) is safe, but only in women who start therapy with CD4 counts below 250. Elective cesarean section is sometimes used to further reduce the risk of transmission to the baby, but it's only necessary if the viral load is detectable at the time of delivery.

If your partner is HIV-negative, you should be on ART with an undetectable load before trying to conceive naturally, to protect him from infection. Short of that, you can use artificial insemination, either performed by a physician or at home using the "turkey baster" approach, in which the partner's semen is squirted into the vagina using a syringe to avoid intercourse. HIV-negative male partners could consider taking PrEP (Questions 13, 86) while trying to conceive, though many experts (including me) think this is overkill if your viral load is undetectable.

HIV-positive women who want to get pregnant should talk to their provider and to an obstetrician-gynecologist with HIV expertise. There are many other issues to discuss besides ART, including safe conception, planning the delivery, breastfeeding, and medical care for the baby, just to name a few.

Pregnancy is a realistic option for HIV-positive women now that we can treat HIV effectively and prevent women passing it to the baby.

Rose's comment:

My dream was always to have a big family, but I felt funny talking to medical providers about having more children because I was positive. My second child was infected because I didn't know I was positive during my pregnancy. My next child was negative because I took antiretroviral therapy, but I was scared to have more children, so I had my tubes tied. After I remarried, I realized I wanted a child with my husband. I started talking to my providers about pregnancy. Getting my tubes untied wasn't easy, but I finally found a fertility doctor who agreed to do it.

Then we had to talk about how to get pregnant without putting my HIV-negative husband at risk. We used the "turkey baster" method, which is artificial insemination done at home. I got pregnant within 3 months. Since I was taking antiretroviral therapy and had an undetectable viral load, I knew that there was very little risk of having another infected baby. I'm a great mom, and I plan on being around for my family for a long time.

77. How can I father a child with an HIV-negative woman?

Conception is a little more complicated when the male partner is positive, because male-to-female transmission is more common than the reverse. Having an undetectable viral load on ART is the most important thing you can do to prevent transmission, and many believe it eliminates the risk entirely, though there are still some theoretical concerns.

Sperm washing

A technique in which sperm are separated from semen to lower the risk of HIV transmission to a woman during conception.

Before we had the ability to fully suppress the viral load—and before we knew how effective it was at preventing transmission—some couples used **sperm washing**, which involves separating sperm from semen and inseminating the HIV-negative woman only with the sperm. The procedure is effective, but available only at a few medical centers and is very expensive.

If you're not comfortable relying entirely on the prevention benefits of an undetectable viral load, there are some additional things that can be done to reduce the risk even further. Intercourse can be timed with the most fertile part of the woman's cycle using home ovulation tests. In addition, the woman can consider using pre-exposure prophylaxis (PrEP) around the time of attempted conception (Question 13). For this, you'll need a prescription and the advice of an expert.

If *both* partners are infected, this is much less of an issue. The HIV status of the father is irrelevant as far as the baby goes, because an infant can only be infected by its mother.

78. What if my child is HIV positive?

A thorough discussion of HIV in children is beyond the scope of this book, which is written for HIV-positive adults. Children and adolescents can be infected either through **mother-to-child transmission** during late pregnancy, labor, or breastfeeding, or through the usual types of transmission (sex or drug use).

Fortunately, mother-to-child transmission has become rare in the United States because of the routine testing of pregnant women and the use of ART during pregnancy. Diagnosing babies is complicated because they carry the mother's HIV antibodies for up to 18 months, regardless of whether they're truly infected.

Mother-to-child transmission

Transmission of HIV from mother to infant during late pregnancy, labor, or breastfeeding.

25

Polymerase chain reaction (PCR)

A laboratory technique used to detect or quantify the DNA or RNA of an infectious organism for diagnostic purposes.

Without treatment, many HIV-positive babies can get sick within the first year of life.

Because the standard blood tests aren't helpful, **polymerase chain reaction** (**PCR**) testing of the blood is used to find the virus itself. Also, the CD4 counts that indicate immunosuppression in children under 5 are higher than those in older children and adults.

Without treatment, many HIV-positive babies can get sick within the first year of life. More often, they may do well initially for several years, not becoming ill until they enter pre-school or grade school. Untreated HIV-positive children may not gain weight or grow normally, and they may have neurologic problems that can cause delayed mental development, poor school performance, or cerebral palsy.

Treatment of children is similar to treatment of adults. However, not all drugs come in forms that kids can swallow, and there aren't as many studies on the treatment of children as there are for adults.

HIV-positive adolescents can be especially challenging... even more challenging than adolescents *without* HIV infection! Issues such as adherence, stigma, discrimination, disclosure, depression, substance abuse, and the prevention of further transmission can be especially daunting at this stage of life. HIV-positive adolescents need to be treated by providers who are experts both in HIV infection and adolescent medicine.

Rose's comment:

I found out I was infected when my daughter tested positive 2 months after she was born. It was only then that I learned that the man I was married to was at high risk. When I found out my daughter was infected, my own health care didn't matter; all I cared about was her. My doctors left me with the impression that she would die soon, which I refused to accept. I used myself as the guinea pig, trying medicines first before I let the doctors use them on her. In 1996, the new cocktails changed both our lives.

My CD4 count was 33 and my viral load was sky-high. All that changed on the cocktail, and my daughter responded beautifully as well. I knew then that we were both going to live. My daughter—the one who was "going to die soon"— is now 19 years old, has an undetectable viral load, and is starting her third year of college!

Diagnosing babies is complicated because they carry the mother's HIV antibodies for up to 18 months, regardless of whether they're truly infected.

WOMEN'S ISSUES, PREGNANCY, AND CHILDREN

PART TWELVE

Coinfection

What if I also have hepatitis C?

What if I also have hepatitis B?

How do I prevent cervical and anal cancer?

More...

79. What if I also have hepatitis C?

"**Coinfection**" with both HIV and hepatitis C virus (HCV) is common, especially among injection drug users, because both viruses are easily passed from one person to another with shared needles or syringes. HCV can also be transmitted sexually, though not as easily as HIV and the hepatitis B virus (HBV). We're now seeing a lot of sexually transmitted HCV among gay and bisexual men, usually a result of rough or poorly lubricated receptive anal sex or "fisting." HCV is a common cause of severe liver disease, including **cirrhosis** (liver scarring) and **hepatocellular carcinoma** (**hepatoma**, or **liver cancer**). Now that people aren't dying of AIDS as often, HCV has become an increasingly important cause of death among HIV-positive people.

Untreated HIV infection can make hepatitis C get worse more rapidly. If you're coinfected with HIV and HCV, it's possible that ART will slow the progression of your hepatitis, though that's still somewhat controversial. You should get vaccinated against the hepatitis A and B viruses if you're not already immune, because those viruses can cause more severe disease in people with HCV infection. Finally, don't drink alcohol. Alcohol use, even in moderation, is a big risk factor for HCV progression.

But unlike HIV and hepatitis B, hepatitis C can be now be *cured*, and easily at that! The dreaded **interferon** is no longer necessary, and in most cases, a mere 2–3 months of therapy, sometimes with no more than a single pill per day, can lead to cure in close to 100% of people. As I write this, the only difficult thing about treating hepatitis C is getting these expensive drugs paid for by insurance companies, Medicaid, and **Medicare**. They're often demanding proof of cirrhosis or severe fibrosis before they'll agree to pay for the drugs. I predict that things will improve as competition for this lucrative marketplace increases, prices decline, and it becomes clear that waiting for severe liver disease to cure hepatitis C has no medical or ethical justification.

If your HCV is being treated by someone other than your HIV provider, make sure they communicate with each other. Some of the HCV drugs interact with antiretroviral medications. You may have to switch to a different ART regimen during treatment for HCV.

It would be ludicrous for me to go into detail about the treatment of hepatitis C at this point, because recommendations seem to change every few months. Let's just say that the news is *great*, and getting better all the time. If I had to pick the most important change in this book from the last edition to his one, hepatitis C treatment and cure would win hands down!

Now that people aren't dying of AIDS as often, HCV has become an increasingly important cause of death among HIV-positive people.

COINFECTION

80. What if I also have hepatitis B?

It's not unusual to be infected with both HIV and the hepatitis B virus (HBV), since both are spread in the same way (sex and blood exposure). Most people who get infected with HBV clear the infection on their own, sometimes after getting sick with hepatitis, but sometimes without ever knowing they were infected. However, others never clear the infection and go on to develop chronic HBV infection, which can lead to chronic hepatitis, cirrhosis, or liver cancer. HIV-positive people are more likely to develop chronic hepatitis B than HIV-negative people.

People who have both HIV and HBV should be treated for both infections at the same time.

HBsAg

A blood test to diagnose acute or chronic hepatitis B. A positive result means there is active hepatitis, but it doesn't distinguish between acute and chronic hepatitis.

HBsAb

A blood test to determine immunity to hepatitis B. A positive result means you're immune to the hepatitis B virus either because of prior infection or vaccination.

Everyone with HIV infection should be tested for HBV, and vice versa. A negative hepatitis B surface antigen (**HBsAg**) generally means you're not infected, though there are rare exceptions. A positive hepatitis B surface antibody (**HBsAb**) means you've been exposed and are immune. If your antibody is negative, you should be vaccinated with a series of three shots. If your surface antibody and antigen are negative but your core antibody (HBcAb or anti-HBc IgG) is positive, you should still be checked for chronic hepatitis with an HBV DNA (the rare exception I spoke of). If that's negative, you should be vaccinated. As with all vaccines, you're more likely to respond to the vaccine if you wait until after you've responded to HIV therapy.

People who have both HIV and HBV should always be treated for both infections at the same time, because some HIV drugs are also active against HBV. Trying to treat just one without causing resistance in the other is difficult and involves taking less desirable medications. The easiest way to treat HIV/HBV coinfection is with an ART combination that contains tenofovir and either emtricitabine or lamivudine. For now, that usually means taking *Atripla, Complera, Stribild,* or a combination of *Truvada* plus a third drug. Lamivudine (3TC, *Epivir,* and contained in *Epzicom, Combivir, Trizivir, Triumeq*) is also active against both HIV and HBV, but unless it's given with tenofovir, resistance will develop. For example, a regimen like *Triumeq* would not be adequate for someone infected with hepatitis B because it contains lamivudine without tenofovir. People who can't take tenofovir can use entecavir (*Baraclude*) in its place.

Stopping HBV drugs can lead to a dangerous flare of hepatitis. People with chronic HBV infection should also get checked periodically for cirrhosis and liver cancer with a CT scan or ultrasound of the liver and the **alpha-fetoprotein (AFP)** blood test.

81. How do I prevent cervical and anal cancer?

Both cervical and anal cancer are caused by human papillomavirus (HPV), a sexually transmitted virus that first causes changes in the cells of the cervix and anus (**dysplasia**) that can later turn into cancer. HPV infection is common, and so is dysplasia. Fortunately, anal and cervical *cancer* are much less common and can be prevented.

The cervical Pap smear is a routine test for women to look for cervical dysplasia. HIV-positive women should get a Pap smear regularly—at least once a year. An abnormal Pap smear is evaluated by **colposcopy**, where abnormal areas can be looked at more closely and biopsied. High-grade lesions can then be treated with minor surgery.

Because **anal dysplasia** is also caused by HPV, involves similar cells, and can also progress to cancer, many experts diagnose and treat anal dysplasia like they do cervical dysplasia, though the evidence is not as strong. That's now possible using an anal Pap smear and **high-resolution anoscopy (HRA)**, the anal equivalent of colposcopy. An anal Pap smear is a simple procedure: a wet swab is inserted in the anus and twisted around on its way out. But it doesn't make sense to do anal Pap smears unless there's someone trained to follow-up the abnormal results with HRA, to biopsy suspicion lesions, and to treat high-grade lesions. Screening for anal dysplasia is mostly done in men who have had sex with

COINFECTION

Alpha-fetoprotein (AFP)

A blood test used to look for liver cancer.

Dysplasia

Abnormal development or growth of tissues, organs, or cells.

Colposcopy

A procedure used to more closely examine the cervix for dysplasia due to HPV infection in women who have had abnormal Pap smears.

Anal dysplasia

Abnormal cells in the anus caused by HPV. If left untreated, it can progress to anal cancer.

High-resolution anoscopy (HRA)

A procedure used to more closely examine the lining of the anus for dysplasia due to HPV infection in people who have had abnormal anal Pap smears.

men and in women, especially women who have cervical dysplasia or anal or genital warts. Straight men can have anal dysplasia too, even straight men who've never had sex with a man, so some argue that we should be doing this test in everybody.

There are now effective vaccines to prevent HPV infection, especially the strains that cause cancer (Question 26). It's approved for men and women up to the age of 26, but is best used in children or adolescents before they become sexually active. If you have children and you're not vaccinating them because you think they'll grow up to be celibate monks and nuns, think again! Young HIV-positive people should be vaccinated, and maybe even older people, though it's hard to get it paid for above the age of 26.

PART THIRTEEN

Mental Health and Substance Abuse

How do I know if I'm depressed?

What should I do if I'm depressed?

What are the risks of using drugs if I'm positive?

More…

82. How do I know if I'm depressed?

HIV-positive people who are depressed may assume they're just having a normal response to being positive. But depression, in the true medical sense of the word, is *never* "normal." People often describe themselves as being "depressed" when what they *really* mean is that they're sad, disappointed, angry, worried, or demoralized—perfectly normal responses to the bad things that happen to all of us in life. Depression, on the other hand, is not a *normal* response to life's misfortunes. Some people can be depressed for no obvious reason when everything's going well objectively, while others experience the sufferings of Job without ever being depressed. While depression can be triggered by life events in people who are prone to it, the fact that you're depressed has more to do with brain chemistry than external circumstances.

People who are depressed feel sad, empty, hollow, hopeless, and isolated. Activities and people they once enjoyed no longer bring pleasure.

People who are depressed feel sad, empty, hollow, hopeless, and isolated. Activities and people they once enjoyed no longer bring pleasure. They may lose interest in sex, work, hobbies, friends, and family. They see no light at the end of the tunnel—the future looks bleak. They may have insomnia or they may sleep too much. They may lose their appetite for food or overeat. They may abuse drugs or alcohol or engage in high-risk sex because they provide momentary relief. Symptoms can include fatigue, weight loss (or gain), memory loss, and headache.

In contrast, people who are experiencing normal coping problems—dealing with an HIV diagnosis, for example—may feel sad, stressed, angry, or worried, but they understand that they'll get through it, and they can be "cheered up" or distracted by keeping busy or by being with friends, or engaging in activities they enjoy.

If my description of depression rings true to you, talk to your medical provider immediately. Depression is a dangerous but highly treatable condition. It's also one of the biggest risk factors for poor adherence with antiretroviral medications—another reason to take it seriously.

Depression is a dangerous but highly treatable condition.

Rose's comment:

I knew I was depressed when I stopped wanting to get up or to clean my house. I lost interest in my children's schools or being in the PTA. I isolated myself and was often tearful or angry. Everything was dark, and everything about me was dark. I stopped paying bills, and I didn't care about my appearance. Of course, I never should have waited until things got that bad. If it ever happened again, I'd know what to look for and would get help sooner.

83. What should I do if I'm depressed?

If you view depression as a normal emotion, a sign of weakness, or a character flaw, you're unlikely to get the help you need. Think of depression as though it were pneumonia. You *might* get better on your own, but it won't be pleasant. It could take a long time. It *could* even kill you. With treatment, things can get better quickly.

The best way to treat depression is to take **antidepressants**—drugs that restore the normal balance of chemicals in your brain, which have become out of balance while you're depressed. There are many antidepressants available. They all work to treat depression but have different side effects. Some antidepressants are sedating, which can be helpful for people with insomnia.

Antidepressants
Drugs used to treat depression.

MENTAL HEALTH AND SUBSTANCE ABUSE

Others can perk you up if you're fatigued or sleeping too much. Some antidepressants can cause sexual side effects, especially delayed orgasm. (Then again, there's nothing like untreated depression to take away sex drive and destroy sexual performance!) Most antidepressants also help control anxiety and obsessive thoughts.

When you take an antidepressant, don't expect sudden or dramatic changes. It can take 2 to 4 weeks before you start to notice a difference. The point isn't to change your personality or to make you ecstatically happy. The point of antidepressants is to make you feel like yourself again. Antidepressants won't change the circumstances of your life, but they can help you cope with those circumstances. They're not habit forming—they can be tapered and stopped when you no longer need them. If you don't tolerate the first drug you try, don't give up. Switch to a drug with a different side effect profile.

The best way to treat depression is to take anti-depressants— drugs that restore the balance of chemicals in your brain that are out of balance when you're depressed.

Counseling and psychotherapy are not a substitute for medications, because in the depths of depression, talking doesn't do much good. Talk therapy becomes useful as you start to get better—it helps you return to life, to deal with issues that might have contributed to your depression, and to keep you healthy after you get better. Psychotherapy is also great for people who aren't depressed but are having problems coping with life circumstances.

Rose's comment:

I was afraid to talk about my depression to Joel (my provider) because back then he was still one of those "white coat guys" that I didn't trust. But I started talking to other people in the waiting room at the clinic, and I realized I wasn't alone—other people had been through this before. When I finally talked to Joel about my depression, he started me on an antidepressant. I slowly began to feel better, and then I realized just how bad I'd let things get. It took about 30 days before I got my energy back and was myself again. The experience also taught me that I could talk to Joel about these things and that he would listen and care. It's very important to have a provider you can talk to.

84. What are the risks of using drugs if I'm positive?

HIV-positive people often assume that drug use is bad for them because it lowers their CD4 count and increases their viral load, but that's not the reason to stay away from drugs. (I wish we could say that "good, clean living" would keep HIV under control, but life isn't fair, and the virus doesn't care what you do.) Still, there are plenty of great reasons to stay away from drugs.

First, there are the medical dangers of the drugs themselves. Cocaine causes heart attacks and mental illness. Heroin injection can lead to serious infections of the heart valves, bones, and joints. Methamphetamine can destroy your teeth, your brain, your relationships, your career, and your life. All three are addictive. It's hard to come up with too many dire warnings about the dangers of marijuana, but even its advocates admit that regular use can make you dumb and lazy, and there's now some evidence that it could increase the risk of mental illness later in life. There is evidence that *Aspergillus*, a fungus that can cause dangerous infections in people with very low CD4 counts, can live in marijuana leaves and can be inhaled. (If you smoke dope and have a low CD4 count, we used to recommend microwaving the joint to kill the fungus. Please don't ask me which setting to use or for how long—those studies will never be done!)

Aspergillus

A fungus that causes aspergillosis, a potentially serious infection involving the lungs that can occur in people with very advanced HIV disease.

Drugs can also interact with your HIV medications. Drug companies don't typically study interactions between their drugs and illegal substances, but there is evidence that people have been harmed by taking "club drugs," such as MDMA (Ecstasy) and ketamine, along with antiretrovirals, for example.

Drug use can increase your risk of getting other infections or of spreading HIV to others. If you've got a drug problem, get treatment before you start ART.

Drug use can increase your risk of getting other infections or of spreading HIV to others. Being high lowers your inhibitions and clouds your judgment, allowing you to take risks that you wouldn't otherwise take, putting you at risk for sexually transmitted diseases, including syphilis (Question 89). Injection is especially risky, since it can spread HIV, hepatitis C, and other bloodborne infections.

Finally, studies show that active drug users are less likely to take ART correctly, putting them at risk of drug resistance and losing treatment options. If you've got a drug problem and starting ART isn't urgent, get treatment before you start. Don't wait until you've messed up and developed drug resistance.

Ultimately, the best reason to stay away from drugs is to keep yourself physically and mentally healthy so you'll have the upper hand against HIV infection.

PART FOURTEEN

Relationships, Sexuality, and Prevention

How and when should I disclose my
HIV status to partners?

How can I have safe sex?

What should I know about
sexually transmitted infections?

More…

85. How and when should I disclose my HIV status to partners?

Being HIV-positive doesn't mean you can't have intimate relationships or sex, but it does complicate things since you have to deal with revealing your HIV status to partners and protecting those who are negative from becoming infected.

The issue of disclosure can be a thorny one. Some argue that disclosure isn't necessary if you're practicing safe sex. They point out that everyone knows the risks and should be protecting themselves, regardless of what their partners say—or don't say—about their status. There are also situations where disclosure is unrealistic. Anonymous sex taking place in a bathhouse or dark alley rarely involves a "How do you do?" much less a detailed exchange of medical information. Then again, someone having sex in that environment should assume a high level of risk and take the appropriate precautions.

Disclosure becomes especially important when you're dating or starting a new relationship. Some deal with this by dating only HIV-positive partners. That simplifies things, but it's not possible for everyone. Disclosing your status to a negative partner can sometimes be a deal breaker, resulting not only in rejection but also—in the worst-case scenario—the risk that your new "ex" may share your information with others. For that reason, many choose to wait until there's mutual affection, trust, and a sense that the relationship is going somewhere.

The problem is that the longer you wait, the more likely your new partner will feel betrayed when you finally disclose your status, especially if the relationship has already become sexual. If you're positive and your goal is to be in a relationship, you may have to take things slower than we're used to these days. Get to know and trust your partner first, talk about your HIV status later, and *then* have sex. If this process takes a while, remember that in Jane Austen novels, couples didn't even use first names until the engagement was announced, and holding gloved hands was evidence that things had progressed to an advanced level of intimacy!

Rose's comment:

Disclosing your status isn't easy, especially to a partner. I sat him down and just blurted out that I was positive. He asked me how it happened, and I explained that I'd been infected by my first husband. I don't know which scared him more, my HIV or the fact that my tubes were tied, but he ran. I thought I'd never see him again. But he was back 2 weeks later. He said he wanted to learn more, and I started educating him about HIV. We talked about condom use, and I told him condoms should be mandatory in any relationship because of HIV and other sexually transmitted infection. We built our relationship from there, and now we've been married for over 8 years.

86. How do I have safe sex?

There is no sexual activity that is guaranteed to transmit HIV infection, and there's at least *some* risk involved in most activities—at least the most popular ones. I can't give you odds or percentages, since the risk depends not only on what you're doing, but on how you're doing it and your viral load. The risk is *dramatically* reduced if the viral load is undetectable. It's hard to promise that the risk is *zero*, because you can't prove a negative, but in two large studies looking at "discordant couples" (couples in which one is positive and the other is negative), we have seen *no* cases of transmission when the positive partner has an undetectable viral load. Being on effective ART is probably *the* most effective way to prevent transmission if you're going to have sex.

Here are some general comments about the "riskiness" of the more common sexual activities, assuming the viral load is detectable and condoms aren't being used:

- *Anal and vaginal intercourse.* If the positive partner is on top, this is the highest-risk activity. A condom reduces the risk dramatically if it doesn't break. The risk is much lower if the positive partner is on the bottom. That's because the lining of the anus and vagina is made of **mucosal cells**, which can be infected, whereas the penis is almost completely covered by skin, which can't. However, a man can still get infected from being on top. The risk is higher if he's uncircumcised or has herpes, syphilis, or other open sores on his penis. The risk of spreading both HIV and the hepatitis C virus increases if there's bleeding during sex.

- *Oral sex.* HIV can be transmitted by getting a positive person's preseminal fluid ("pre-cum"), semen ("cum"), vaginal fluid, or menstrual blood in the mouth. (It has nothing to do with swallowing, because the stomach is an inhospitable place for viruses to survive.) The risk is higher if the gums are in bad shape. If the positive partner is giving oral sex to the negative partner, there's essentially no risk of HIV transmission, though other STIs can be spread that way.

- *Oral-anal sex ("rimming").* You won't spread HIV this way, but the person doing the rimming could get hepatitis A or a bacterial or parasitic gastrointestinal infection.

Mucosal cells

Cells that line the internal organs and body orifices, such as the mouth, nostrils, anus, and genital area.

- *Mutual masturbation.* This is very safe as long as you don't have open cuts or sores on the hands and keep fluids out of the mouth and eyes.
- *"Water sports."* Urine is a safe bodily fluid.
- *Kissing, hugging, cuddling, massage.* All safe.

87. What if my partner is negative?

Let's assume that disclosure is out of the way (Question 85). You're positive and your negative partner knows it. What next?

It's your responsibility to make sure you never infect *anyone,* including your negative partner. "This infection stops with me" are words to live by. Of course, HIV-negative adults should be aware of the risks and should be protecting themselves as well. Unfortunately, that approach hasn't been working, and the U.S. epidemic continues to grow at a rate of about 50,000 new cases per year. Prevention experts are now changing the prevention message to focus on those who are positive—people who know better than anyone how important it is to prevent transmission and who must bear most of the responsibility for not spreading the infection.

Uninfected people sometimes make crazy choices and stupid decisions. Some may seem perfectly willing to put themselves at risk of infection. It's the moral obligation of the positive partner not to cooperate with that kind of self-destructive behavior, to ensure that their HIV is never transmitted. "Every man for himself" is not a philosophy that we should want to live by. We live in a community and should watch out for each other.

RELATIONSHIPS, SEXUALITY, AND PREVENTION

The most important thing you can do to prevent transmission to a negative partner is to maintain an undetectable viral load on ART, the most effective form of prevention we have. As I've already said, that may be all you need, especially if you've been "undetectable" for years and get your labs checked regularly. But for some HIV-negative people, that may not be enough, which is their choice. They may still want to use condoms, especially for high-risk activities or to prevent other sexually transmitted infections. In some cases, they may choose to use PrEP for greater piece of mind. On a societal level, we can't afford to treat both HIV-positive people *and* their HIV-negative partners with antiretroviral medications to prevent transmission, but I probably wouldn't refuse PrEP to someone who insisted on it and had a way to pay for it. For more on the relative risk of various sexual activities, see Question 86.

88. What if my partner and I are both positive?

Being with a positive partner eliminates concerns about new HIV transmission, but there are still reasons to consider protected sex, including avoidance of other sexually transmitted infections (Question 89) and **superinfection**. We know that HIV-positive people can be superinfected with additional strains of virus. There have been some welldocumented cases, which also explains why there are **recombinant strains** of HIV in the world (viruses that are combinations of two or more **subtypes**). Superinfection can cause a rise in viral load and a drop in CD4 count, similar to what happens with initial infection. You could also become superinfected with a drug-resistant strain of virus, especially if you were taking drugs that your partner's virus was resistant to.

Superinfection

Reinfection with a new strain of HIV in someone who has already been infected.

Recombinant strains

Strains of HIV that are combinations of two or more other strains.

Subtypes

In the case of HIV, groups of related viruses, also called "clades" or "subclades." Most HIV-positive people in the United States are infected with subtype B, but there are many other subtypes throughout the world.

Superinfection can cause a rise in viral load and a drop in CD4 count, similar to what happens with initial infection.

Proving superinfection requires the kind of testing that isn't readily available through commercial labs, so we don't know how often it occurs. It's probably not common, and there's evidence that it happens mostly to people who have only been infected for a few years, but not in those with longstanding infection. Two people with undetectable viral loads don't have to worry about superinfection.

When talking to my positive patients about sex with other positive partners, I recommend condoms with casual partners, mainly to prevent sexually transmitted infections. In steady relationships, the decision to abandon condoms will depend on how long each partner has been infected, whether they're monogamous, their viral loads, whether either partner has resistant virus, whether or not they're likely to be infected with the same strain (did one get infected by the other?), and whether there are other transmittable infections to consider, such as hepatitis C virus.

89. What should I know about sexually transmitted infections?

Becoming positive doesn't mean you can stop worrying about sexually transmitted infections (STIs). You've got the Big One, but there are others to be avoided.

Syphilis can be worse in people with HIV infection. It can progress more rapidly if it's not treated. It's more likely to infect the nervous system, and can affect your vision and hearing. The blood tests we use to monitor your response to syphilis treatment can be harder to interpret and can take longer to become negative than in HIV-negative people. If you're HIV-positive, you should

Syphilis

A sexually transmitted infection caused by *Treponema pallidum*, a bacterium, that can cause anal, genital, or mouth lesions (primary syphilis), fever, rash, and hepatitis (secondary syphilis), or infection of the brain, spinal fluid, eyes, or ears (neurosyphilis). It can also be dormant, causing no symptoms (latent syphilis).

be checked for syphilis, and the test should be repeated at least once a year—more often if you're sexually active with multiple partners.

Gonorrhea

A sexually transmitted infection caused by the bacterium Neisseria gonorrhoeae.

Chlamydia

A sexually transmitted infection caused by Chlamydia trachomatis.

Lymphogranuloma venereum (LGV)

A sexually transmitted infection caused by *Chlamydia*.

Proctitis

Infection or inflammation of the rectum.

Gonorrhea and **chlamydia** are common infections that can infect the urethra of the penis, the cervix, the anus, and the throat. Gonorrhea has become resistant to standard oral antibiotics and must now be treated with an injection. (In fact, if things keep going the way they're going with drug resistance, you may soon need intravenous therapy to treat gonorrhea). HIV-positive men should be checked for gonorrhea and chlamydia with a urine test and also with anal and/or throat swabs if they're having anal and/or oral sex; women should be tested at the time of their routine pelvic exam. A different type of chlamydial infection, **lymphogranuloma venereum** (**LGV**) sometimes causes anal and rectal infections (**proctitis**) in gay men. It tends to be more severe than standard chlamydia and takes longer to treat. I hear gay men tell me they've been "tested for STDs," but all they've had is a syphilis blood test and a urine test, which only looks for gonorrhea and chlamydia in the urethra of the penis. If you're having oral and anal sex and no one has swabbed your throat and butt, you've haven't really been tested.

Genital herpes, usually caused by herpes simplex virus type 2 (HSV-2), causes painful blisters and shallow ulcers on the genitals, around the anus, or on the skin. The infection persists for life and can recur, especially in people with low CD4 counts. ART can help, but outbreaks should be treated with an anti-herpes medication, such as acyclovir, famciclovir, or valacyclovir. If you're having frequent outbreaks, you should take one of those medications daily, which not only prevents herpes flares, but also the risk of herpes (and possibly HIV) transmission.

Human papillomavirus (HPV) infection is discussed in Questions 26 and 81. There are other STIs that I haven't discussed but that are also best avoided.

PART FIFTEEN

Living with HIV Infection

What foods and water are safe?

Should I take vitamins or supplements?

Can I travel abroad?

More…

90. What foods and water are safe?

There are few foods you should *avoid* eating because of HIV infection, but there are some guidelines to follow, especially if your CD4 count is low. Avoid undercooked meat, especially if your *Toxoplasma* antibody is negative (Question 56). Avoid raw eggs, undercooked poultry, unpasteurized milk or fruit juices, and raw sprouts. Hard cheeses (like cheddar) are safer than soft cheeses (like brie, feta, Camembert, or Mexican cheeses), which may contain *Listeria*, a bacterium that can cause meningitis (though not often). Avoiding raw shellfish is a good idea, but if you can't resist a raw oyster, make sure you're immune to hepatitis A (Question 26). Some doctors recommend avoiding sushi, but that seems cruel and extreme to me since the parasites you can get from sushi aren't worse if you have HIV than if you don't. Be careful not to "cross-contaminate" food when you're preparing it. For good food safety tips, check out www.foodsafety.gov.

Cryptosporidium is a parasite that can be passed from person to person or ingested in contaminated water.

What *should* you eat? Healthy food, preferably *real* food: food that you or someone else cooks from original, pronounceable ingredients. Eat fresh fruits and vegetables—with every meal, every day. Starches should be brown, not white—the white, refined starches just get turned into sugar. Speaking of sugar, think of dessert as a special treat, not a daily course. To gain weight, eat more. To lose weight, eat less. Break the rules once in a while, but not every day. When you *do* break the rules, break them without guilt. Finally, before you develop too many rigid dietary rules or restrictions, remember that eating is not a form of medical therapy but one of life's great pleasures. *Bon appetit!*

What about water? For most HIV-positive people, tap water is perfectly safe. If you're young and not familiar with the term "tap water," it refers to a plentiful, healthy beverage that people used to drink *directly from faucets and drinking fountains without charge*, but that has been replaced by an expensive, bottled version that I call "tap water from a city you don't live in." How millions of gullible Americans were duped into voluntarily handing over money to large corporations for something that is still free is a great mystery, but it happened—the discarded plastic evidence of it is everywhere.

The best reasons to pay for water are if your tap water tastes bad, is known to be of bad quality, or if you like it fizzy. Otherwise, tap water is fine for most people. If your CD4 count is below 100, be aware of the risk of **cryptosporidiosis**. *Cryptosporidium* is a parasite that can be passed from person to person or ingested in contaminated water. Tap water is usually safe, but there have been occasional outbreaks when the water supply becomes contaminated. You can protect yourself by filtering tap water through a 100-micron filter. Bottled water is OK, too, but only if the company filters it in the same way, which is not guaranteed.

Cryptosporidiosis

Diarrhea caused by *Cryptosporidium*, a parasite that can be found in contaminated water or transmitted from person to person.

91. Should I take vitamins or supplements?

If you've just read the previous answer, you can probably guess how I'm going to answer this one. A healthy diet should provide you with all the nutrients you need. If your diet consists of fast food and sodas, then taking a multivitamin is a good idea. Vitamin supplements are good for you if you're vitamin deficient, but there's little evidence that they help you if you're already eating well. In fact, studies are finding that some vitamins and herbs can be harmful when taken out of their "natural habitat"—say an apple or a piece of broccoli—and put into a tablet or capsule. A standard multivitamin is harmless and cheap, but I hate to see people spending lots of their hard-earned cash on the latest supplement touted on the web or at the health food store: money they could be spending on eating good food. If you're going to take vitamins anyway, don't spend a lot of money. Compare ingredients and buy the cheap, generic stuff.

The only exception is vitamin D, which is probably the only vitamin supplement that still gets good press these days. Vitamin D deficiency is common in both HIV-negative and HIV-positive people, and may be worse if you're taking efavirenz (*Sustiva*, *Atripla*). I generally recommend supplementation to all my patients. For those with osteopenia or osteoposis, calcium is also important—preferably through your diet but with supplements if you're not getting enough.

In no way am I a nutritional nihilist. I believe very strongly in nutrition, which is best achieved by eating well.

92. Can I still drink alcohol?

The answer depends on whether it would have been OK for you to drink if you were HIV-negative. HIV infection itself has very little to do with it. First, let's talk about who should *not* drink:

1. People with chronic hepatitis B or C shouldn't drink because it can make the hepatitis worse and increase the risk of cirrhosis (see Questions 79 and 80). After you've been cured of hepatitis C, you can consider drinking in moderation, provided you don't have cirrhosis.

2. Alcoholics shouldn't drink because few are capable of drinking in moderation. Excessive alcohol consumption is bad for just about every organ in your body. It is especially bad for your liver, which may already be stressed by some of the medications we use to treat HIV infection. There are other conditions that can be caused by both alcohol abuse and by either HIV infection or ART, including neuropathy, dementia, blood disorders, heart problems, and pancreatitis, just to name a few. Why increase your risk? Finally, people who are drunk are lousy medication takers, and we've already talked about what happens when you don't take your medications (Question 29). If you're wondering whether you're an alcoholic, there's a good chance you are. If alcohol has repeatedly caused problems with your work, relationships, or criminal or driving record, if you can't control your drinking, if other people think you drink too much, if you feel guilty or lie about your drinking, if you wake up hungover or shaky until you get an eye-opener, then you've got a problem, one that needs to be addressed *before* you start HIV therapy.

If you can drink in moderation and have no medical reason to avoid alcohol, then drinking is OK with HIV and with all HIV medications. Alcohol does not interfere with the activity of the medications or increase their toxicity, as long as you're not overdoing it. Keep it down to a maximum of two drinks per day: two glasses of wine, two beers, or two ounces of hard liquor. (And if you don't drink all week, that doesn't mean you can have 14 drinks on Friday night!)

If you can drink in moderation and have no medical reason to avoid alcohol, then drinking is OK with HIV and with HIV medications.

93. Can I travel abroad?

Yes, but there are a few things to consider, especially if you're going to a resource-limited country where there are bugs you wouldn't normally come in contact with. If your CD4 count is over 200, the risk is about the same as it would be for anyone else. But if your count is low, especially less than 50, then you might reconsider your destination or wait until your count is higher.

Typhoid vaccine

A vaccine to prevent typhoid fever, a bacterial infection of the blood caused by *Salmonella typhi*, sometimes acquired by travelers to developing countries.

Yellow fever

A serious disease caused by yellow fever virus, which is transmitted by mosquitoes and sometimes acquired by travelers to parts of Africa or Latin America.

The CDC website (www.cdc.gov/travel/) has excellent country-specific information about precautions and vaccinations. HIV-positive people with low CD4 counts (less than 200) should generally avoid vaccines that contain live viruses or bacteria. This is especially true for oral **typhoid vaccine** (get the injectable vaccine instead). If **yellow fever** vaccine is required and your CD4 count is low, consider going to Orlando rather than Ouagadougou. Getting the vaccine is fine if you have a high CD4 count and there's a definite risk of yellow fever where you're going. Make sure you've had a tetanus booster in the last 10 years and have been vaccinated against hepatitis A and B if you're not already immune (Question 25). Take the usual precautions to avoid travelers' diarrhea, and talk to your doctor about bringing an antibiotic along to treat it if it happens.

HIV-positive people should generally avoid vaccines that contain live viruses or bacteria.

No matter where you're going, make sure you have enough meds for the entire trip and then some. Plan ahead for cancelled or delayed flights—they happen! Bring the original bottles to avoid problems at the airport, and carry them on the plane rather than checking them in your luggage.

Finally, consider taking the names of some HIV doctors or clinics in the areas you're traveling to, especially if your medical condition is complex or if you'll be away for a long time.

Bon voyage!

94. Can I have pets?

Don't drown Kitty in the river just because you're HIV-positive! You can still have pets if you follow a few simple precautions. And remember that most of the concerns and precautions pertain to people with low CD4 counts.

If possible, stay away from very young animals (less than 6 months old), and avoid contact with sick animals. Pets with diarrhea should get checked for bugs in their feces that could be passed on to you. Wash your hands well after handling your pets and before eating.

Cats can carry *Toxoplasma gondii*, the parasite that causes toxoplasmosis (Question 56), which you get from eating cat poop. *"But I don't eat cat poop!"* you protest. These things can happen, usually if you've been changing a litter box and get it on your hands and then in your mouth. Assuming you're not already infected (find out whether you have a positive *Toxoplasma* antibody), the best solution is to get someone else to change the litter box. If you and Kitty live alone together, then wear gloves, wash your hands, and change the box every day because it's harder to get toxo from fresh poop. Indoor kitties are safer than the outdoor prowlers. Take the same precautions with gardening, too.

Cats can also transmit *Bartonella*, the bacterium that causes cat-scratch disease in children as well as bacillary angiomatosis (a skin disease) and **peliosis hepatis** (an

Peliosis hepatis

An uncommon liver infection caused by *Bartonella*.

infection of the liver) in HIV-positive people. Older cats are safer than young ones. Don't play rough with Kitty. Fortunately these are uncommon, treatable conditions— not a justification for de-clawing as a preventative measure. Sorry, but you can't use your HIV status as an excuse to save your sofa!

Reptiles, chicks, and ducklings can carry *Salmonella,* a bacterium that causes diarrhea and other problems, especially in HIV-positive people. Wash well after handling Mr. Lizard or consider trading him in for a different animal. There have also been reports of *Salmonella* in common pet treats, so don't share them with your animals.

What about dogs? I have *nothing* bad to say about dogs.

95. Can I still exercise?

You can and you should! Mainly because it's a healthy way to live, and it's important to maintain your overall health if you're HIV-positive. But there are some reasons to exercise that are specific to HIV as well:

1. Some of the older antiretroviral drugs can cause fat accumulation, insulin resistance, and elevations in cholesterol and triglycerides (Questions 43 and 46), which in turn can increase the risk of heart disease, and some people who are now on newer agents are stuck with these problems from drugs they took in the past. Aerobic exercise helps to reverse all of those conditions.

2. Although we don't know the cause, we're seeing loss of bone density in people with HIV infection (Question 50). Exercise, especially resistance exercise, can help to maintain bone density.

3. Some of the older antiretroviral drugs caused lipoatrophy (fat loss) involving the legs, arms, and buttocks (Question 46). Resistance training can increase the muscle mass in these areas, which can help to compensate for the loss in fat. (Note that vigorous aerobic exercise, while great for fat accumulation, may make lipoatrophy worse... there's no justice!)

4. HIV-positive people are at greater risk for depression. Exercise is a great natural antidepressant.

If you're not used to exercising, start slow. Walk more. Take the stairs. Park in the far corner of the lot. If you're a fair-weather walker, join a gym. Don't do the same type of exercise each day, but mix it up so you don't get bored. Exercise with a friend, or listen to music or a recorded book, my personal favorite way to spend a tedious hour on the exercise bicycle. A slug-like existence may be more likely to kill you than HIV, so *don't be a slug!*

96. What are advance directives?

Can I be blunt? *Everybody dies.* Whether you have HIV, some other chronic disease, or are the picture of health, you will someday take your last breath. Before we had effective treatment for HIV disease, an untimely death from AIDS was a virtual certainty. In those days, I spent a lot of time talking to my patients about death and dying and helping them make end-of-life decisions. Today, we spend more time talking about life, old age, and retirement, but I still encourage my patients (and friends and family members) to make plans and discuss their wishes about death and dying with the people who matter. The best time to think about these things is when you're healthy and have no immediate plans to leave the planet.

What kind of medical care would you want if you were sick and unable to make decisions for yourself? Would you want life-sustaining measures—to be resuscitated with **CPR** or to be put on a breathing machine in the intensive care unit—if the chances of recovery were low? Would you want any treatment at all, including artificial feeding, if you had a terminal illness? Who would you choose to make medical decisions for you?

If you know the answers to these questions, you need **advance directives**—legal documents that make your wishes known to others in case you can't speak for yourself. A **living will** is a legal document that lets you spell out the medical treatments and life-sustaining measures you would want or not want if you were unable to make those decisions for yourself. A living will is important, but it's not enough because it doesn't cover every decision that might need to be made. It's even more important to choose the person who would make medical decisions for you if you couldn't make them for yourself. If that person is your legally recognized spouse, then you're covered, because your spouse is automatically your next of kin. But if you want decisions to be made by an unmarried partner, a friend, or a different family member, then you need to appoint that person using a **durable power of attorney for health care**, a legal document that trumps next-of-kin rules, and your living will too, for that matter. This document also allows your partner or friend to visit you in the hospital if visitation is otherwise limited to immediate family members. The person you appoint should be aware of your wishes

CPR

Cardiopulmonary resuscitation. Procedures used to try to revive someone whose heart has stopped and/or has stopped breathing.

Advance directives

Legal documents that allow you to make decisions about end-of-life care ahead of time.

Living will

A legal document that allows you to state which medical procedures and life-sustaining measures you would want if you were no longer able to make decisions for yourself.

Durable power of attorney for health care

A legal document that allows you to authorize someone else to make medical decisions on your behalf if you lose the ability to make decisions for yourself.

in advance—including what's in your living will—and should agree to act in accordance with those wishes.

Everyone should have these documents. You don't need a lawyer—the forms are available online and in most clinics and hospitals. Give a copy to your provider and to the person you've named as your decision maker.

You should also have a will, especially if you want your belongings to go to someone other than your immediate family members. Whether you'll need a lawyer to draw up a will depends on how complex your finances and your wishes are. Simple wills can be drafted using software programs.

No one likes to think or talk about dying, but the consequences of not having advance directives can be tragic. Make your wishes known, and make them count!

PART SIXTEEN

Questions for Those Who Still Have Questions

What about the theory that HIV doesn't cause AIDS?

Isn't it true that drug companies are withholding the cure to make money?

What's the state of the global epidemic?

More...

97. *What about the theory that HIV doesn't cause AIDS?*

In the early years of the AIDS epidemic, shortly after the discovery of HIV, a few scientists questioned whether AIDS was really caused by HIV infection. They proposed a number of alternative explanations, suggesting that AIDS was caused by drug abuse and zidovudine (in the developed world) and malnutrition (in the developing world). These scientists argued that **Koch's postulates** had not been fulfilled and warned that antiretroviral therapy, rather than saving lives, was prematurely ending them.

If their hypothesis was far-fetched in the late-1980s, it's complete lunacy today. Koch's postulates have been fulfilled many times over. We now have a solid and ever-growing understanding of how HIV infects human cells, damages the immune system, and causes AIDS. The life-saving effects of ART have been well established by countless clinical trials, large observational studies, and data from large populations. It was no accident that the death rate from AIDS declined by 50% in the year after HAART was introduced!

The few so-called "scientists" who cling to their discredited hypotheses have forgotten one of the fundamental principles of science: You have to be able to admit that you might be *wrong*. Their dwindling followers (most have either died prematurely or have come to their senses and started therapy before it was too late) now treat "HIV denialism" more as a religious cult than as a scientific hypothesis. These nut-jobs would be amusing if it weren't for their influence. They affected the policies of the South African government for many years, resulting in years of preventable deaths and new infections,

Koch's postulates

The four criteria needed to prove that a microbe or organism is the cause of a disease. The postulates are: 1) The organism must be found in all animals suffering from the disease but should not be found in healthy animals 2) the organism must be isolated from a diseased animal and grown in pure culture; 3) he cultured organism should cause disease when introduced into a healthy animal; and 4) he organism must be reisolated from the experimentally infected animal.

and they have influenced gullible people to refuse an effective treatment for a fatal disease. They will have a lot to atone for when they arrive at the Pearly Gates.

98. Isn't it true that drug companies are withholding the cure to make money?

This is a popular point of view among conspiracy theorists and those with contempt for drug companies, but a little rational thought should put this myth to rest:

1. It's no surprise that we haven't yet cured HIV infection. The difficulty of finding a cure is discussed in Question 14.

2. People who develop therapies at drug companies are scientists. They're motivated by the things that motivate scientists everywhere else: publication in prestigious journals, the respect of their colleagues, Nobel Prizes, TV interviews, getting funding to do more research, and the knowledge that their work has made a difference to humankind. No scientist who discovers the cure for AIDS is going to keep quiet about it, even if ordered to do so by an evil, profit-hungry CEO!

3. Drug companies are competitive. If they're onto something big, their competitors can't be far behind. No company strives to be the *second* company with The Cure. If a company had a cure, you'd have heard about it!

4. A cure for AIDS will be highly profitable. Sure, there's profit in lifetime therapy, too, but it's shared among multiple competing drug companies and doesn't last forever. Drugs go off patent and get replaced by generics; they fall out of favor as they're replaced by newer and better agents.

Look at hepatitis C, where a cure costs around over $80,000. A cure for HIV is likely to be even more expensive. Shed no tears for the pharmaceutical industry when we have a cure. It will be highly lucrative for the company that develops it.

5. *Most* conspiracy theories are wrong.

99. How do we know HIV wasn't created in a lab?

This popular conspiracy theory gives *way* too much credit to the science of bygone generations. HIV first infected humans in the first half of the 20th century. We have proof of human infection dating back to the 1950s, and it probably became a human disease several decades before that. The idea that such a complex virus could be created by scientists today is far-fetched enough, but to think that it could have been invented 80 years ago is preposterous.

Throughout history, there have been infamous examples of abuse of the human race by science and medicine, but the deliberate creation of the HIV epidemic is not one of them.

Few of those who believe in this theory think it was just an innocent scientific experiment gone wrong. Instead, they think it was part of a well orchestrated plot to rid the country—or the world—of its "undesirable elements": gay men, injection drug users, or minorities...take your pick. But in the 1930s we were worried about poverty; in the 1940s, it was the Germans and Japanese; and in the 1950s and 1960s, it was the communists. No one had the time or resources to think about wiping out gay men and drug users, who were barely on the radar screens of anyone except *other* gay men and drug users.

The fact that the HIV epidemic didn't originate in the developed world—where, as we know, all the Evil Scientists live—doesn't fit well with this theory either.

Because the epidemic began in Africa, you'd have to propose that someone was trying to wipe out all Africans, a strategy that would not have been appreciated by the colonial powers who relied on them for labor and income.

Finally, it's inconceivable that the inventor of such a virus could have planned an epidemic that would target specific groups of people. Its spread among gay men, drug users, and minorities was accidental, and of course it didn't stay confined to those groups. Throughout history, there have been infamous examples of abuse of the human race by science and medicine, but the deliberate creation of the HIV epidemic is *not* one of them.

100. What's the state of the global epidemic?

I've been fairly upbeat in this book, talking about HIV infection as the chronic, manageable disease that it's become. That's because if you're reading this book, you probably live in a place where treatment is available and affordable. It's more challenging to be optimistic about the state of the global epidemic. More than 39 million people have died of AIDS, and more than 35 million are now living with HIV infection, most of them in recource-limited countries, especially in sub-Saharan Africa. AIDS killed about 1.5 million people in 2013. It has wiped out hard-earned economic and healthcare gains in many developing countries, drastically reducing life expectancy and creating millions of orphans, whose prognosis is grim regardless of their HIV status. The epidemic threatens to cause economic, social, and civil collapse in countries where large proportions of the population—including the leaders, teachers, doctors, and civil servants—are infected and dying.

The news hasn't been *all* bad. In about 2000, the developed world finally recognized that it couldn't go on ignoring the devastation in the poorer parts of the world, and money began flowing from the government, private, and philanthropic sectors to provide life-saving treatment for people throughout the world, or at least in those countries where there was a political will to deal with the AIDS epidemic. Generic drugs made treatment more affordable.

The global financial crisis threatened the progress that had been made, and although the economy has now improved in the United States, the commitment of our country and the other wealthy countries of the world depends very much on the whims of politicians. In addition, the treatment being offered in most of the world would still be considered second-class by our standards. Viral load and resistance testing are often too expensive, and fewer drugs are available, so options are limited if the first regimen fails. Most importantly, the number of new infections is far higher than the number of people being started on treatment—despite our progress, we fall further behind each year.

I can't begin to do justice to these issues here in this final answer. My hope is that HIV-positive people who read this will see themselves as part of a larger global community, one in which there are enormous inequities but great promise and hope. Our planet hasn't faced such a crisis in its history. How we confront it will determine our future and what those who live in the future say about us. We have the resources, the intelligence, and the creativity to solve this problem; all we need is the will, the compassion, and the right sense of priorities.

Additional Resources

This book is by no means comprehensive. If you've read it cover to cover, you've just dipped your toe in the water. There are many good sources of information for HIV-positive people, most of it on the Internet. I invite you start with my own interactive, question-and-answer forum at www.hivforum.tumblr.com. If that's not enough, here are some more sites to keep you busy:

Websites
- *AIDS.gov.* Basic information on HIV and on U.S. government strategy and programs: http://aids.gov/.
- *AIDSinfo.* A site of the U.S. Department of Health and Human Services (HHS), where you can find the latest treatment guidelines, drug information, and news about clinical trials: www.aidsinfo.nih.gov.

- *AIDS InfoNet.* A project of the New Mexico AIDS Education and Training Center that provides information on HIV treatment and prevention in multiple languages: www.aidsinfonet.org.
- *AIDSmeds.* A good source of information about HIV treatment: www.aidsmeds.com.
- *AIDS Treatment News.* A newsletter for HIV-positive people: http://aidsnews.blogspot.com.
- *American Academy of HIV Medicine.* You can find information about HIV providers in your area: www.aahivm.org.
- *AmfAR (American Foundation for AIDS Research).* Provides information on HIV, including research developments: www.amfar.org.
- *AVERT.* Domestic and international HIV information, news, and stories: www.avert.org.
- *BETA (Bulletin of Experimental Treatments for AIDS).* A bulletin published by the San Francisco AIDS Foundation covering new developments in HIV therapy: www.sfaf.org/hiv-info/hot-topics/beta/.
- *The Body.* A patient-oriented site that provides updated information, coverage of new scientific findings, and answers to users' questions: www.thebody.com.
- *CDC National Center for HIV/AIDS, Viral Hepatitis, STD, and TB Prevention.* CDC website with basic HIV information and data on the U.S. epidemic: www.cdc.gov/nchhstp/.

- *Clinical Trials.gov.* A source of up-to-date information about federally and privately supported clinical research studies, including trials of HIV therapies: www.clinicaltrials.gov.

- *GMHC (Gay Men's Health Crisis).* A New York–based, patient-oriented website that provides basic HIV information and news: www.gmhc.org.

- *HIVandHepatitis.com.* Scientific updates: www.hivandhepatitis.com.

- *HIV InSite* HIV information from the University of California, San Francisco: http://hivinsite.ucsf.edu/.

- *National AIDS Treatment Advocacy Project (NATAP).* Excellent source of information on new scientific data on HIV and hepatitis C, including studies presented at scientific conferences: www.natap.org.

- *New York State Department of Health AIDS Institute.* Provides general information about HIV/AIDS: www.health.state.ny.us/diseases/aids/.

- *POZ.* An online and print magazine for HIV-positive people: www.poz.com.

- *TPAN.* A magazine for HIV-positive people, that includes updates on drug development and scientific developments: www.tpan.com.

- *Project Inform.* An organization that provides updated information about HIV treatment: www.projectinform.org.

A

Abscesses: Collections of pus (infectious organisms and white blood cells) in the skin ("boil") or other parts of the body.

Acquired immunodeficiency syndrome: *See* **AIDS**.

Acute retroviral syndrome (ARS): A constellation of symptoms, such as fever, rash, and swollen lymph nodes, that most people experience during primary infection, shortly after they're infected.

Acyclovir: A drug used to treat herpes simplex and varicella zoster virus.

ADAP: *See* **AIDS Drug Assistance Program**.

Adherence: The term used to refer to a patient's behavior with respect to following treatment recommendations, including taking medications, keeping medical appointments, etc.

Adrenal glands: Glands in the abdomen that produce cortisol, a steroid hormone that is essential to many bodily functions, including the response to stress.

Adrenal insufficiency: A deficiency in the amount of cortisol produced by the adrenal gland.

Advance directives: Legal documents that allow you to make decisions about end-of-life care ahead of time. *See* **Living will and Durable power of attorney for health care**.

Advanced HIV infection: The most advanced stage of HIV infection, usually in people with CD4 counts below 50 or 100.

Aerosolized pentamidine: *See* **Pentamidine**.

AIDS: Acquired immunodeficiency syndrome, a more advanced stage of HIV infection, defined by having a CD4 count below 200 or one of a list of AIDS indicator conditions (see Table 1).

AIDS case definition: The criteria used by the Centers for Disease Control and Prevention (CDC) to classify someone as having AIDS (*see* **AIDS**).

AIDS-defining condition: *See* **AIDS indicator condition**.

AIDS Drug Assistance Program (ADAP): A federally funded program that provides antiretroviral medications and other HIV-related medications to those who have no other way to pay for them. The programs are administered by the states, and coverage varies from state to state.

AIDS-indicator condition (or AIDS-defining condition): One of a list of conditions, including opportunistic infections and malignancies, that is used by the CDC to determine who has AIDS (see Table 1).

AIDS-related complex (ARC): An old term, no longer in use, for the stage of HIV disease in which people have symptoms but have not yet developed AIDS. Now referred to as "symptomatic HIV infection."

AIDS service organization (ASO): An organization that provides services to people with HIV infection.

Alpha-fetoprotein (AFP): A blood test used to look for liver cancer.

Alternative medicine: The use of a non-standard medical treatment in place of standard therapy.

Amphotericin B: An intravenous drug used to treat serious fungal infections.

Anal cancer: Cancer of the anus caused by human papillomavirus (HPV).

Anal dysplasia: Abnormal cells in the anus caused by human papillomavirus (HPV). If left untreated, it can progress to anal cancer.

Anal Pap smear: A diagnostic test to screen for anal dysplasia. Also called "anal cytology."

Anemia: A deficiency of red blood cells, usually diagnosed by a low hemoglobin or hematocrit on a complete blood count.

Angular cheilitis: Cracking of the corners of the lips, sometimes caused by *Candida*.

Anoscopy: See **High resolution anoscopy**.

Anti-HBs: *See* **HBsAb**.

Antibodies: Proteins used by the immune system to fight infection. Antibodies are formed after exposure to antigens—foreign substances such as viruses or bacteria.

Antidepressant: Drugs used to treat depression.

Antigens: Proteins from organisms, such as bacteria or viruses, that stimulate an immune response.

Antiretroviral therapy (ART): Drug therapy that stops HIV from replicating and improves the function of the immune system.

Anti-CMV IgG antibody test: A blood test used to look for infection with CMV.

Anti-*Toxoplasma* IgG antibody test: A blood test used to look for exposure to the *Toxoplasma* parasite.

Aphthous ulcers: Painful ulcers in the mouth (aphthous stomatitis) or esophagus (aphthous esophagitis) that can occur in people with HIV. The cause is unknown.

ARC: *See* **AIDS-related complex.**

ART: *See* **Antiretroviral therapy.**

Aseptic meningitis: Meningitis that is not caused by a bacterium that can be grown in culture. Can be caused by viruses (including HIV during acute retroviral syndrome) or drugs.

Aspergillus: A fungus that causes aspergillosis, a potentially serious infection involving the lungs that can occur in people with very advanced HIV disease.

Asymptomatic HIV infection: An early stage of HIV infection in which infected people have a positive test but no symptoms.

Atovaquone: A drug used to treat or prevent PCP, sold under the trade name *Mepron*.

Attachment: The first stage of entry, in which the virus binds to the CD4 receptor. Attachment inhibitors would block this step, though none are currently approved.

Avascular necrosis: Painful joint damage caused by osteonecrosis, usually affecting the hips but sometimes the shoulders.

Azithromycin: An antibiotic that can be used to treat or prevent MAC as well as some bacterial lung infections.

B

Bacillary angiomatosis: A bacterial disease of the skin caused by *Bartonella*, which causes raised purple lesions on the skin; sometimes confused with Kaposi's sarcoma.

Bacterial vaginosis: A bacterial infection of the vagina that causes vaginal discharge.

Bactrim: *See* **Trimethoprim-sulfamethoxazole.**

Bartonella: A bacterium that can cause skin disease (bacillary angiomatosis) or liver disease (peliosis hepatis) in people with HIV.

Bell's palsy: A paralysis of one side of the face that can be caused by a variety of infections, including acute HIV infection.

Benzodiazepine: A class of drugs used to treat anxiety and insomnia. Diazepam (*Valium*) and alprazolam (*Xanax*) are well known examples. The drugs can be habit-forming and can interact with some antiretroviral drugs.

Bilirubin: A pigment produced in the liver. When bilirubin levels get too high, the skin and eyes can turn yellow ("jaundice" or "icterus"). Elevated bilirubin can be caused by hepatitis or by two antiretroviral drugs: indinavir (*Crixivan*) or atazanavir (*Reyataz*).

Biopsy: A procedure in which a piece of tissue is removed, either with a needle through the skin, through a scope placed in the lungs or gastrointestinal tract, or by a surgical procedure. The specimen is then examined under the microscope and/or submitted for culture to make a diagnosis.

Blip: A single detectable viral load with undetectable viral loads before and after.

Boosted protease inhibitors: These combine a protease inhibitor (PI) with cobicistat or with a low dose of ritonavir (*Norvir*), another PI that is used only to increase drug levels and prolong the half-life of other PIs.

Bronchitis: An infection of the bronchi (airways), usually caused by a viral infection, often after a common cold.

Bronchoscopy: A diagnostic procedure in which a flexible tube is inserted into the lungs through the mouth (under sedation) so that samples or biopsies can be taken.

Bronchospasm: The tendency of the bronchi (airways in the lung) to constrict (narrow), causing shortness of breath or cough. This can be chronic (in patients with asthma, for example) or temporary, following an upper respiratory infection.

Burkitt's lymphoma: A type of lymphoma that is seen more frequently in people with HIV infection but is less common than non-Hodgkin's lymphoma (NHL).

C

Candida: A fungus (yeast) that can cause thrush, esophagitis, and vaginitis in people with HIV infection.

Candidiasis: An infection caused by *Candida*, a common yeast.

Case manager: A person who helps coordinate your medical care, provides referrals for needed services, and determines whether you qualify for any assistance or entitlement programs.

CBC: *See* **Complete blood count**.

CCR5: *See* **Coreceptor**.

CCR5 antagonist: A drug that blocks CCR5.

CD4 cell: *See* **CD4 lymphocyte**.

CD4 count (or **CD4 cell count**): A lab test that measures the number of CD4 cells in the blood (expressed as number of cells per cubic millimeter). The CD4 count is the most important measure of immunosuppression and is the most important indicator of the need for treatment.

CD4 lymphocyte (or **CD4 cell**, or **T-helper cell**): A type of lymphocyte (a type of white blood cell) that can be infected by HIV. CD4 cells fight certain infections and cancers. The number of CD4 cells (CD4 count) declines with untreated HIV infection, which leads to immunosuppression.

CD4 percent: The percentage of lymphocytes that are CD4 cells. The CD4 percent is provided whenever a CD4 count is ordered and provides additional information about the state of the immune system.

CD4 receptor: A protein on the surface of the CD4 cell that the virus attaches to before entering the cell.

CD8 cells (or **CD8 lymphocytes**, or **T-suppressor cells**): Another type of lymphocyte affected by HIV infection. Measuring CD8 cells is not necessary, as the CD8 count is not used to make treatment decisions.

CD8 lymphocytes: *See* **CD8 cells**.

CDC: *See* **Centers for Disease Control and Prevention**.

Cellular immune system: The part of the immune system most directly affected by HIV infection. It controls a variety of bacterial, viral, fungal, and parasitic infections.

Centers for Disease Control and Prevention (CDC): A branch of the federal government, within the U.S. Department of Health and Human Services (HHS) that is charged with tracking, preventing, and controlling health problems in the United States, including infectious diseases such as HIV.

Cervical cancer: Cancer of the cervix (the mouth of the uterus) caused by human papillomavirus (HPV).

Cervical dysplasia: Abnormal cells of the cervix, the mouth of the uterus, caused by human papillomavirus (HPV). If left untreated, it can progress to cervical cancer.

Chemokines: *See* **Coreceptors**.

Chickenpox: *See* **Varicella zoster virus**.

Chlamydia: A sexually transmitted infection caused by *Chlamydia trachomatis*.

Cholesterol: A substance found in body tissues and the blood. Cholesterol is ingested (in meat or animal products) and also manufactured by the body. Cholesterol levels are measured by blood tests.

Cirrhosis: A form of permanent liver damage caused by alcoholism or chronic hepatitis.

Clarithromycin: An antibiotic that can be used to treat or prevent MAC as well as some bacterial lung infections.

Clinical trial: A study in which a treatment for a medical condition is tested in human volunteers to determine the safety and/or effectiveness of the treatment. In the case of HIV, this could include the study of investigational or approved drugs. In a randomized trial, two or more treatments are compared, and the treatment is selected by random chance. In a double-blind trial, neither the subject nor the investigator knows which treatment the subject is receiving. In a placebo-controlled trial, a drug is compared against an inactive substance that is identical in appearance. In a multicenter trial, the same trial is conducted simultaneously at multiple centers, sometimes in multiple countries. Phase I trials evaluate safety and drug levels and help to determine a dose range in a small number of volunteers who may be HIV-positive or negative. Phase II trials are conducted in a larger

number of subjects, looking at both safety and effectiveness, often of several doses of the medication. Phase III trials are large studies conducted at multiple sites that are designed to find out whether the treatment is effective and to collect more safety information. Phase IV trials occur after a treatment is already approved to find out more about its effectiveness, safety, and the best way to use it.

Clotrimazole troches: Antifungal lozenges used to treat thrush.

CMV: *See* **Cytomegalovirus**.

Coccidioidomycosis ("cocci"): A disease caused by **Coccidioides immitis**, a fungus found mostly in the deserts and valleys of the southwestern United States and northern Mexico. It can cause lung disease, meningitis, and infection of other organs.

Cocktail: An outdated term for an antiretroviral regimen (combination of antiretroviral drugs).

Coinfection: The combination of two infections, such as HIV plus either hepatitis B virus or hepatitis C virus.

Colitis: Infection or inflammation of the colon (large intestine).

Colonization: The presence in the body of microorganisms (viruses, bacteria, etc.) that are not causing symptoms or disease.

Colonoscopy: A medical procedure in which a flexible scope is inserted into the rectum and colon through the anus, while the patient is sedated, in order to look for abnormalities and take biopsies.

Colposcopy: A procedure used to more closely examine the cervix for dysplasia due to human papillomavirus (HPV) infection in women who have had abnormal Pap smears.

Combination antiretroviral therapy (cART): Another term for "HAART."

Combination therapy: The use of more than one antiretroviral drug to suppress HIV infection.

Complementary and alternative medicine (CAM): Medical products or treatments that are not standard of care (*see* **Alternative medicine** and **Complementary medicine**).

Complementary medicine: The use of a non-standard medical treatment in addition to standard therapy.

Complete blood count (CBC): A standard blood test that measures the red and white blood cell counts, hematocrit, hemoglobin, and platelet count.

Compliance: *See* **Adherence**.

Comprehensive chemistry panel: A standard blood test that measures kidney function, looks for evidence of liver disease, assesses nutritional status, and looks for electrolyte (sodium, potassium) abnormalities.

Coreceptors (or chemokines): Proteins on the surface of the CD4 cell and other cells that the virus binds to after attaching to the CD4 receptor but before entering the cell. There are two coreceptors: CCR5 and CXCR4.

Cortisol: The steroid hormone produced by the adrenal gland essential to many bodily functions, including the response to stress.

Cotrimoxazole: *See* **Trimethoprim-sulfamethoxazole**.

CPR: Cardiopulmonary resuscitation. Procedures used to try to revive someone whose heart has stopped and/or has stopped breathing.

Cross-resistance: Resistance to one drug that results in resistance to other drugs, usually in the same class.

Cryptococcal antigen: A lab test performed on either blood or spinal fluid used to diagnose cryptococcal meningitis.

Cryptococcal meningitis: Meningitis (infection of the spinal fluid and spinal cord lining) caused by *Cryptococcus*.

Cryptococcus: A fungus or yeast that is a common cause of meningitis in people with HIV infection.

Cryptosporidiosis: Diarrhea caused by *Cryptosporidium*, a parasite that can be found in contaminated water or transmitted from person to person.

Cryptosporidium: The parasite that causes cryptosporidiosis, which can cause chronic diarrhea in immuno-suppressed people. The organism can be found in contaminated water or transmitted from person to person.

Cushing's syndrome: Excessive cortisol levels either because of overproduction by the adrenal glands or use of steroid medications.

CXCR4: *See* **Coreceptors**.

Cytomegalovirus (CMV): A virus that can infect the eyes, the gastrointestinal tract, the liver, and the nervous system in people with advanced HIV. The most common cause of retinitis (infection of the back of the eye).

D

Dapsone: A drug used to treat or prevent PCP and to prevent toxoplasmosis.

Daraprim: *See* **Pyrimethamine**.

Delta 32 deletion: A genetic condition resulting in the absence of CCR5 coreceptor on the CD4 cell.

Individuals who are heterozygous for this deletion (the mutation is present in only one copy of the gene) can be infected by HIV but progress more slowly. Those who are homozygous (the mutation is present in both copies of the gene) cannot be infected by R5 virus, the most common form of circulating HIV.

Detectable: A word used to describe a viral load that is high enough to be measured by a viral load test. A detectable viral load is one that is above 20 to 75, depending on the test being used.

Detoxification: The removal of toxic substances from the body. An important function of the liver and kidneys.

Diabetes: A disorder resulting in elevated amounts of glucose (sugar) in the blood and urine.

Directly observed therapy (DOT): A program in which treatment is given to a patient directly by a healthcare professional, at home or in a clinic, in order to ensure that it's taken. Most common with treatment for tuberculosis but sometimes used for HIV therapy.

Disclosure: The process of revealing your HIV status to others.

Drug classes: Categories or groups of HIV drugs that are classified based on the way the drugs work and the stage of the viral life cycle that they target.

Drug holiday: An old term for an interruption in therapy, usually when the decision was made by the patient.

dT: *See* **Tetanus toxoid**.

Durable power of attorney for health care: A legal document that allows you to authorize someone else to make medical decisions on your behalf if you lose the ability to make decisions for yourself.

Dysphagia: Difficulty swallowing.

Dysplasia: Abnormal development or growth of tissues, organs, or cells.

E

EBV: *See* **Epstein-Barr virus**.

EIA: *See* **Enzyme-linked immunoassay**.

ELISA: *See* **Enzyme-linked immunoassay**.

Elite controllers: HIV-infected people whose CD4 counts remain high and whose viral loads are undetectable without treatment.

Encephalitis: An infection of the brain.

Endoscopy: A medical procedure in which a flexible tube is inserted into the esophagus and stomach through the mouth, while the patient is sedated, in order to take samples or biopsies or to treat a variety of conditions.

Enzyme-linked immunoassay (ELISA or EIA): Traditionally, the initial antibody test used to diagnosed HIV infection. Positive tests were confirmed with Western blot assays.

Enteritis: Infection or inflammation of the small intestines.

Entry: The process by which HIV enters human cells.

Entry inhibitors: Drugs that block entry of the virus into the CD4 cell.

Envelope: The outer surface of the HIV virus.

Enzymes: Proteins that carry out a biological function. Examples of enzymes carried by HIV include reverse transcriptase, integrase, and protease. Each plays a role in allowing the virus to reproduce, and each is a target for antiretroviral therapy.

Epidemic: The appearance of new cases of disease (especially an infectious disease) in a human population at a higher rate than would be expected.

Epstein-Barr virus (EBV): A herpesvirus that causes infectious mononucleosis ("mono"), oral hairy leukoplakia, and some lymphomas.

Erythematous candidiasis: An infection of the mouth caused by *Candida* in which the roof of the mouth (palate) becomes red and sometimes painful.

Esophagitis: Infection or inflammation of the esophagus.

Esophagus: The tube that connects the mouth and throat to the stomach.

Ethambutol: A drug used to treat MAC and TB, in combination with other drugs.

F

Failure: Loss of activity of ART. Includes virologic failure (detectable viral load on therapy), immunologic failure (falling CD4 count on therapy), and clinical failure (worsening symptoms on therapy).

Famciclovir: A drug used to treat herpes simplex and varicella zoster virus.

Family Medical Leave Act (FMLA): A federal law that allows people to take time off work without fear of termination or loss of benefits to deal with their own serious or chronic medical problems or those of their family members. People who need this protection must file paperwork with their employers in advance.

Fasting glucose: Measures blood glucose levels after hours without food.

Fat accumulation (or lipohypertrophy): A component of the "lipodystrophy syndrome" in which fat accumulates in abnormal parts of the body, such as inside the abdomen, around the neck, in the breasts, or on the upper back at the base of the neck ("buffalo hump").

Flu: *See* **Influenza**.

Fluconazole: A drug used to treat fungal infections.

Flucytosine (5FC): A drug used to treat fungal infections, usually in combination with amphotericin.

FMLA: *See* **Family Medical Leave Act**.

Folinic acid: *See* **Leucovorin**.

Folliculitis: Infection of the hair follicles and skin around them.

Fourth-generation HIV tests: HIV tests that detect both antigen and antibody, allowing them to detect HIV infection sooner after infection than older antibody tests.

Fusion: The final stage of viral entry in which the envelope of the virus fuses (merges) with the membrane of the cell, allowing entry of the virus into the cells. A fusion inhibitor blocks this process.

G

Gastrointestinal: Relating to the GI tract: esophagus, stomach, small intestines, colon, and rectum.

Gastritis: Infection or inflammation of the stomach.

Genotype tests: In HIV, a type of resistance test that looks for specific resistance mutations known to cause resistance to antiretroviral drugs.

Gonorrhea: A sexually transmitted infection caused by the bacterium *Neisseria gonorrhoeae*.

gp120: The part of the envelope (outer surface) of HIV that binds to receptors on the surface of the CD4 cell, allowing entry into the cell.

Guillain-Barré syndrome: Progressive muscle paralysis starting in the legs and moving upward, sometimes seen during acute retroviral syndrome.

H

HAART: *See* **Highly active antiretroviral therapy**.

Half-life: The amount of time it takes for the blood levels of a drug to decline by 50% after the last dose. Drugs with longer half-lives remain in the blood longer and can be taken less often.

HAV antibody: A blood test for hepatitis A. The IgM antibody tests for acute hepatitis A. The total or IgG antibody tests for prior infection or vaccination.

HBsAb (or anti-HBs): A blood test for hepatitis B. A positive result means you're immune to the hepatitis B virus either because of prior infection or vaccination.

HBsAg: A blood test for hepatitis B. A positive result means there is active hepatitis, but it doesn't distinguish between acute and chronic hepatitis.

HBV DNA: The "viral load" for hepatitis B, used to make the diagnosis in some people with negative HBV antibodies and to monitor response to hepatitis B therapy.

HCV RNA: The "viral load" for hepatitis C, used to confirm the diagnosis in people with a positive HCV antibody, to make the diagnosis in some people with a negative antibody, and to monitor response to hepatitis C therapy.

Hematocrit: A measure of the amount of red blood cells in the blood. (*See* **Complete blood count and Anemia**.)

Hemoglobin: The oxygen-carrying component of red blood cells. Also used as a measure of the amount of red blood cells in the blood. (*See* **Complete blood count** and **Anemia**.)

Hepatic steatosis ("fatty liver"): A buildup of fat in the liver that can be caused by a variety of medical conditions. When caused by antiretroviral agents it is often accompanied by lactic acidosis.

Hepatitis: Inflammation or infection of the liver.

Hepatitis A: A viral infection of the liver caused by hepatitis A virus (HAV). It is spread by ingestion of feces or of food or water contaminated by feces. Unlike hepatitis B and C, hepatitis A never causes chronic infection.

Hepatitis B: A viral infection of the liver caused by hepatitis B virus (HBV). Like HIV, it is spread sexually, through exposure to infected blood or at childbirth. A proportion of people with HBV infection can develop chronic hepatitis and liver disease.

Hepatitis C: A viral infection of the liver caused by hepatitis C virus (HCV). It is spread primarily through exposure to blood (injection drug use or occupational exposures), but can also be transmitted sexually. Hepatitis C commonly causes chronic infection.

Hepatocellular carcinoma (or **hepatoma, or liver cancer**): Cancer of the liver that can be caused by alcoholism or chronic hepatitis.

Hepatoma: *See* **Hepatocellular carcinoma**.

Hepatotoxicity: *See* **Liver toxicity**.

Herpes simplex virus (HSV): A virus that causes painful blisters and ulcers on the lips, genitals, near the anus, or other parts of the skin.

Herpesvirus: A family of viruses that can cause acute infection but that also remain latent in the body and recur. Examples of herpesviruses include herpes simplex virus (HSV-1 and HSV-2), varicella zoster virus (VZV), cytomegalovirus (CMV), Epstein-Barr virus (EBV), and human herpesvirus-8 (HHV-8).

Herpes zoster: *See* **Shingles**.

HHV-8: The virus that causes Kaposi's sarcoma, Castleman's syndrome, and some rare lymphomas. Also called Kaposi's sarcoma–associated herpesvirus (KSHV).

Highly active antiretroviral therapy (HAART): Antiretroviral therapy meant to suppress the viral load to undetectable levels, using a combination of several agents to prevent resistance (now usually just referred to as antiretroviral therapy [ART]).

High-resolution anoscopy (HRA): A procedure used to more closely examine the lining of the anus for dysplasia due to human papillomavirus (HPV) infection in people who have had abnormal anal Pap smears.

Histoplasmosis: A disease caused by *Histoplasma capsulatum*, a fungus found mostly in the Ohio and Mississippi River valleys, which causes lung infection in people with normal immune systems, and infection of the lungs and other organs in people with low CD4 counts.

HIV: Human immunodeficiency virus, the virus that causes HIV infection and AIDS.

HIVAN: *See* **Nephropathy, HIV-associated**.

HIV-1: The most common form of HIV worldwide.

HIV infection (or HIV disease): The name for the disease caused by HIV infection. AIDS is a late stage of HIV infection.

HLA B*5701: A blood test used to predict the likelihood of the abacavir hypersensitivity reaction (HSR). If the test is positive, you shouldn't take abacavir. If it's negative, you're extremely unlikely to develop HSR.

Hodgkin's disease: A type of lymphoma that is more common in people with HIV but is less common than non-Hodgkin's lymphoma (NHL).

Home test: An HIV blood test that can be performed at home.

HPV: *See* **Human papillomavirus**.

HRA: *See* **High-resolution anoscopy**.

HSR: *See* **Hypersensitivity reaction**.

Human herpesvirus-8: *See* **HHV-8**.

Human immunodeficiency virus: *See* **HIV**.

Human papillomavirus (HPV): A sexually transmitted virus that causes abnormal cells (dysplasia) in the cervix, anus, and mouth, which can lead to cancer if not treated.

Humoral immune system: The part of the immune system that uses antibodies to fight infection. It is less affected by HIV infection than the cellular immune system.

Hyperlipidemia: An abnormal elevation of lipids (cholesterol and/or triglycerides) in the blood.

Hypersensitivity reaction (HSR): A reaction, often allergic, to a medication or other substance.

Hypogonadism: A deficiency of testosterone, the male sex hormone.

Hypothyroidism: A deficiency in thyroid hormone.

I

Immune activation: A general stimulation of the immune system that can be caused by a variety of infections, including HIV infection. In the case of HIV, it is thought to cause the decline in CD4 count that occurs with time.

Immune-based therapy: Treatment for HIV infection designed to affect the immune system and its response to the virus, as opposed to standard antiretroviral therapy, which suppresses the virus itself.

Immune system: The system in the body that fights infection.

Immunodeficiency (or immuno-suppression): A state in which the immune system is damaged or impaired, either from birth (congenital immunodeficiency) or acquired, as in HIV infection.

Immune reconstitution inflammatory syndrome (IRIS): A condition that sometimes occurs in people with low CD4 counts who start ART in which the improved immune system reacts to organisms (such as MAC, the TB bacterium, or fungi), causing illness, including fevers, weight loss, swollen lymph nodes, or abscesses.

Indeterminate HIV test: This occurs when the EIA is positive but the Western blot contains some bands that are seen with HIV infection, though not enough to make a diagnosis. This can occur during the process of seroconversion or it can be found in uninfected people, usually for unclear reasons.

Induced sputum: A test used to diagnose PCP or tuberculosis in which patients inhale a saline mist that makes them cough deeply. The sputum specimen is then sent to the lab for analysis. Also called "sputum induction."

Influenza ("flu"): A viral infection caused by influenza virus that causes fever, muscle aches, respiratory symptoms, and gastrointestinal symptoms during winter months and should be prevented by vaccination in the fall. A bad cold is not the flu.

INH: *See* **Isoniazid**.

Insulin resistance: A condition in which the body cannot respond to insulin as well as it should. This applies both to insulin naturally produced by the pancreas and insulin injected as medication. Can lead to high blood sugar or diabetes.

Integrase: A viral enzyme that allows integration (insertion) of viral DNA into human DNA.

Integrase inhibitor: An antiretroviral drug that blocks the integration process.

Integration: The insertion of viral DNA into human DNA in the nucleus of the cell.

Interferon: An injectable medication used in the past to treat hepatitis C and sometimes hepatitis B.

Interferon-gamma releasing assay (IGRA): A blood test used to detect latent infection with the TB bacterium as an alternative to a tuberculin skin test. *QuantiFERON-TB Gold* is the most commonly used IGRA.

IRIS: *See* **Immune reconstitution inflammatory syndrome**.

Isosporiasis: A disease caused by the parasite *Isospora belli*, which causes chronic diarrhea in people with low CD4 counts. Uncommon in the United States and other developed countries.

Isoniazid (INH): A drug used to treat or prevent tuberculosis.

J

JC virus: The cause of progressive multifocal leukoencephalopathy (PML).

K

Kaposi's sarcoma (KS): A tumor caused by a virus that is more common in people with HIV infection, especially gay men. Although it usually affects the skin, KS can also affect other parts of the body, including the gastrointestinal tract and lungs.

Kaposi's sarcoma–associated herpesvirus (KSHV): *See* **HHV-8**.

Kidney biopsy: A procedure in which a piece of a kidney is removed using a needle inserted through the skin in order to find out the cause of kidney disorders.

Koch's postulates: The four criteria needed to prove that a microbe or organism is the cause of a disease. The postulates are: 1) The organism must be found in all animals suffering from the disease but should not be found in healthy animals 2) the organism must be isolated from a

diseased animal and grown in pure culture; 3) the cultured organism should cause disease when introduced into a healthy animal; and 4) the organism must be reisolated from the experimentally infected animal.

KS: *See* **Kaposi's sarcoma**.

KSHV: *See* **Kaposi's sarcoma–associated herpesvirus**.

L

Lactic acidosis: A dangerous build-up of lactic acid (lactate) in the blood, which can be caused by some antiretroviral drugs and also by other medical conditions.

Latency: The ability of HIV to persist in human cells for the lifetime of an infected individual by inserting its DNA into long-lived reservoir cells.

Latency-reversing agents: Drugs being studied in experimental cure strategies that activate HIV-infected resting CD4 cells in order to eliminate the latent reservoir (*see* **Shock and kill**).

Leukopenia: A decrease in the number of white blood cells found in blood.

Leucovorin (folinic acid): A drug used to prevent bone marrow toxicity due to pyrimethamine.

LGV: *See* **Lymphogranuloma venereum**.

Life cycle: In HIV infection, the stages that the virus goes through, starting with its entry into human cells and ending with its replication and the release of new virus particles into the blood.

Lipid panel: A blood test that measures lipid levels in your blood (cholesterol and fats).

Lipoatrophy: Loss of subcutaneous fat (fat under the skin) in the legs, arms, buttocks, and face, caused by some nucleoside analog reverse transcriptase inhibitors (NRTIs).

Lipodystrophy: A general term for changes in body shape and fat distribution caused by some antiretroviral agents. Can include lipoatrophy, fat accumulation, or both.

Lipohypertrophy: *See* **Fat accumulation**.

Listeria: A foodborne bacterium that can cause meningitis and other infections. Although not common, the risk for acquiring *Listeria* is higher in people with HIV.

Liver cancer: *See* **Hepatocellular carcinoma**.

Liver enzymes: *See* **Transaminases**.

Liver toxicity (or **hepatotoxicity**): Damage to the liver caused by medications.

Living will: A legal document that allows you to state which medical procedures and life-sustaining measures you would want if you were no longer able to make decisions for yourself.

Log (logarithm): Another way of expressing viral load results. A viral load of 100,000 is a viral load of five logs; 10,000 is four logs; 1,000 is three logs. A tenfold change in viral load is a one-log change. For example, a drop in viral load from 100,000 to 1,000 is a "two-log drop."

Lumbar puncture: *See* **Spinal tap**.

Lymphadenopathy: Swollen or enlarged lymph nodes ("glands"). (*See also* **Persistent generalized lymphadenopathy**.)

Lymph nodes: Structures of the human body that are part of the immune system, acting as filters that collect and destroy bacteria and viruses.

Lymphocytes: A type of infection-fighting white blood cell. CD4 cells are a type of lymphocyte.

Lymphogranuloma venereum (LGV): A sexually transmitted infection caused by *Chlamydia*.

M

MAC: *See* **Mycobacterium avium complex**.

MAI: *See* **Mycobacterium avium complex**.

Medicaid: An insurance program funded by the federal and state governments that provides coverage for medical care to low-income, uninsured people.

Medicare: A federally funded program to provide medical insurance primarily to the elderly and disabled.

Meningitis: An infection or inflammation of the spinal fluid and the lining of the spinal cord.

Methicillin-resistant *Staphylococcus aureus* (MRSA): A drug-resistant bacterium that traditionally caused serious illness in seriously ill hospitalized patients but that has recently become a common cause of skin disease, including abscesses (community-acquired MRSA).

Microsporidia: A variety of opportunistic parasites that cause chronic diarrhea in people with low CD4 counts.

Migraine headache: A severe headache, often on one side of the head, sometimes accompanied by visual changes or nausea.

Molluscum contagiosum: Flesh-colored bumps or protuberances on the skin that are caused by a poxvirus and can be sexually transmitted.

Mother-to-child transmission: Transmission of HIV from mother to infant during late pregnancy, labor, or breastfeeding.

MRSA: *See* **Methicillin-resistant *Staphylococcus aureus*.**

Mucosal cells: Cells that line the internal organs and body orifices, such as the mouth, nostrils, anus, and genital area.

Mutation: Changes in the normal genetic make-up of an organism due to a mistake that occurs during reproduction. In the case of HIV, some mutations can cause resistance, allowing the virus to replicate in the presence of antiretroviral drugs.

***Mycobacterium avium* complex (MAC)**: A bacterium related to tuberculosis that causes disease in people with advanced HIV disease, including fever, night sweats, weight loss, diarrhea, liver disease, abdominal pain, and anemia. Also known as *Mycobacterium avium intracellulare* (MAI).

Myelitis: Infection or inflammation of the spinal cord.

Myopathy: An inflammation of muscles causing muscle pain and weakness, sometimes seen with acute retroviral syndrome, high-dose zidovudine, or statin drugs used to lower cholesterol.

N

National Institutes of Health (NIH): An agency of the federal government (under the U.S. Department of Health and Human Services) responsible for conducting and funding medical research.

Nephropathy, HIV-associated (HIVAN): A disease of the kidneys caused by HIV infection. It is seen primarily in black patients.

Neuropathy (or peripheral neuropathy): Damage to the nerves resulting in numbness or burning pain, usually in the feet or legs. Can be caused by HIV, some antiretroviral drugs, or other conditions.

Neuropsychological testing: A series of tests, usually performed by a psychologist or neurologist, to assess memory and thinking skills. Can be used to diagnose dementia, or to determine whether someone has depression or dementia.

NHL: *See* **Non-Hodgkin's lymphoma**.

NIH: *See* **National Institutes of Health**.

NNRTIs: *See* **Non-nucleoside reverse transcriptase inhibitors**.

Non-Hodgkin's lymphoma (NHL): The most common type of lymphoma in people with HIV infection.

Non-nucleoside reverse transcriptase inhibitors (NNRTIs): A class of antiretroviral drugs that blocks reverse transcription of viral RNA into DNA by interfering with the activity of reverse transcriptase.

Non-steroidal anti-inflammatory drugs (NSAIDs): Drugs that are commonly used to suppress inflammation and treat pain. Some are available without a prescription.

NRTIs: *See* **Nucleoside analog reverse transcriptase inhibitors**.

NSAIDs: *See* **Non-steroidal anti-inflammatory drugs**.

Nucleoside analog reverse transcriptase inhibitors (NRTIs or "nukes"): A class of antiretroviral drugs that blocks reverse transcription of viral RNA into DNA by mimicking nucleosides, the normal building blocks of DNA.

"Nukes:" *See* **Nucleoside analog reverse transcriptase inhibitors**.

Nystatin: An antifungal mouth rinse used to treat thrush.

O

Odynophagia: Painful swallowing.

OI: *See* **Opportunistic infections**.

Opportunistic infections (OIs): Infections that takes advantage of immunodeficiency. Some opportunistic infections occur *only* in people who are immunosuppressed; others can occur in anyone but are more severe or progressive with immunosuppression.

Oral hairy leukoplakia (OHL): Painless white plaques, or "stripes," on the sides of the tongue caused by Epstein-Barr virus.

Oropharyngeal candidiasis: *Candida* (yeast) infection involving the mouth and throat, including thrush, angular cheilitis, and erythematous candidiasis.

Osteonecrosis: Damage to bones at the large joints. *See* **Avascular necrosis**.

Osteopenia: Loss of bone density ("thinning of the bones").

Osteoporosis: Severe osteopenia, which can lead to bone fractures.

P

Pancreas: An organ in the abdomen that makes insulin and enzymes that help digest food.

Pancreatitis: Inflammation of the pancreas, resulting in abdominal pain, loss of appetite, nausea, and vomiting. Can be fatal.

Pandemic: A global epidemic.

Pap smear: A diagnostic test used to look for cervical dysplasia and cervical cancer. Now also being used to diagnose anal dysplasia (*see* **Anal Pap smear**).

Pathogen: An infectious organism (bacterium, virus, fungus, or parasite) that causes disease.

PCNSL: *See* **Primary central nervous system lymphoma**.

PCP: Used to stand for *Pneumocystis carinii* pneumonia, one of the most common OIs in an HIV-positive patient. It now stands for *Pneumocystis pneumonia*, because of the change in the species name. *See* **Pneumocystis**.

PCR: *See* **Polymerase chain reaction**.

Peliosis hepatis: An uncommon bacterial liver infection caused by *Bartonella*.

Pelvic inflammatory disease (PID): A serious infection of the uterus and fallopian tubes usually caused by sexually transmitted infections, especially gonorrhea and chlamydia.

Pentamidine: A drug used to treat PCP. Aerosolized pentamidine is sometimes used as an inhaled mist to prevent PCP.

Perinatal transmission: *See* **Mother-to-child transmission**.

Peripheral neuropathy: *See* **Neuropathy**.

Pharynx: Throat.

Phenotype test: A type of resistance test that measures the ability of the virus to replicate in varying concentrations of antiretroviral drugs.

PID: *See* **Pelvic inflammatory disease**.

Plasma HIV RNA: *See* **Viral load**.

Platelets: Blood cells that help blood clot. A low platelet count, which can sometimes occur due to HIV infection, can result in easy bleeding or bruising.

PML: *See* **Progressive multifocal leukoencephalopathy**.

Pneumococcal vaccine: Vaccines (Prevnar 13, Pneumovax) recommended for HIV-positive adults to prevent pneumonia caused by the pneumococcus.

Pneumococcus: The common name for *Streptococcus pneumoniae*, a frequent cause of bacterial pneumonia.

Pneumocystis: A fungus (*Pneumocystis jiroveci*) that is a common cause of pneumonia (PCP) in people with HIV infection.

Pneumonia: An infection of the air spaces of the lungs, which can be caused by a variety of infectious organisms.

Polymerase chain reaction (PCR): A laboratory technique used to detect or quantify the DNA or RNA of an infectious organism for diagnostic purposes.

PPD: *See* **Tuberculin skin test**.

Pre-exposure prophylaxis (PrEP): A form of HIV prevention in which antiretroviral medications are taken by HIV-negative individuals to prevent infection.

PrEP: *See* **Pre-exposure prophylaxis**.

Primary central nervous system lymphoma (PCNSL): A lymphoma involving the brain, seen only in people with advanced HIV disease.

Primary HIV infection: The stage of HIV infection that occurs shortly after infection. At this stage, the viral load is very high but antibody tests may be negative or indeterminate. People often have symptoms during this stage (*see* **Acute retroviral syndrome**).

Proctitis: Infection or inflammation of the rectum.

Progressive multifocal leukoencephalopathy (PML): An infection of the brain caused by JC virus, which results in progressive neurologic deterioration.

Prophylaxis: Prevention, usually applied to the use of medications taken to prevent opportunistic infections or to keep them from coming back after they've been treated.

Protease: A viral enzyme that cuts large viral proteins into smaller proteins, which are then used to create new virus particles. A protease inhibitor (PI) is an antiretroviral drug that blocks this process.

Prurigo nodularis: A condition characterized by itchy bumps on the skin, seen more commonly in people with HIV.

Psoriasis: A skin condition that results in dry, scaly, itchy plaques on the skin that can get worse with immunosuppression due to HIV infection.

Purified protein derivative (PPD): *See* **Tuberculin skin test**.

Pyrimethamine: A drug used to treat or prevent PCP or toxoplasmosis.

Q

QuantiFERON-TB Gold: The most commonly used interferon-gamma releasing assay (IGRA), a blood test for latent tuberculosis infection.

R

R5 virus: HIV that enters the CD4 cell using the CCR5 coreceptor. This type of virus can be treated with CCR5 inhibitors. (*See also* **Coreceptor**.)

Radiculitis (radiculopathy): Infection or inflammation of the nerves that emerge from the spinal cord.

Rapid tests: HIV tests that provide an answer within a few minutes, using either blood or saliva. Positive tests must be confirmed with standard serologies.

Reactive airways: *See* **Bronchospasm**.

Recombinant strains: Strains of HIV that are combinations of two or more other strains.

Red blood cell (RBC): Blood cells that carry oxygen to the organs of the body. If you don't have enough of them, you're anemic.

Regimen: A combination of antiretroviral drugs.

Relapse: The return of an illness or disease, usually in someone with a chronic condition.

Replication: The reproduction or multiplication of an organism, including HIV. The replication of HIV is a complex, multi-step process involving infection of a human cell and use of both viral enzymes and human cellular machinery to create new virus particles, which are then released and can infect new cells.

Reservoir: Long-lived human cells that can be infected by HIV, allowing it to persist (remain latent) for the lifetime of the individual. Resting CD4 cells are the best known example, but there are other reservoirs in the human body.

Resistance: The ability of the virus to replicate despite the presence of antiretroviral medications.

Resistance test: A blood test (either a genotype or phenotype) that looks for HIV that is resistant to antiretroviral medications.

Resting CD4 cells: CD4 cells that live a long time and can harbor HIV DNA, which can't be affected by antiretroviral therapy the cell is not replicating, and thus are an important reservoir of latent HIV.

Retinitis: An infection of the retina (the interior surface of the back of the eye), which can lead to blindness if not treated. Most often caused by CMV.

Retrovirus: A virus that contains RNA and that can turn RNA into DNA through reverse transcription using viral enzymes. (*See* **Reverse transcription**.) HIV is a retrovirus.

Reverse transcriptase (RT): An enzyme contained within the HIV virus that can turn viral RNA into DNA so it can be inserted into the DNA of human cells. A reverse transcriptase inhibitor blocks this process.

Reverse transcription: The conversion of viral RNA into DNA by reverse transcriptase. (Normal transcription involves the conversion of DNA into RNA.)

Rifabutin: A drug used to treat or prevent MAC. It is also used as an alternative to rifampin to treat tuberculosis.

Rifampin: A drug used to treat tuberculosis and some other bacterial infections.

RNA: Ribonucleic acid, the genetic material of the HIV virus. Viral RNA gets turned into DNA by reverse transcriptase, and the viral DNA then gets inserted into the DNA of human cells. DNA is later transcribed back into RNA, which in turn gets translated into the proteins that are used to make new virus particles.

RT: *See* **Reverse transcriptase**.

Ryan White Care Act: A government-funded program that provides money on a state or local level to provide care for uninsured people with HIV infection.

S

Salmonella: A group of bacteria that can cause severe diarrhea, fever, and bloodstream infections.

Scabies: An itchy skin condition caused by a mite that burrows under the skin and can be spread to others by close contact.

Seborrheic dermatitis: A common skin condition causing flakiness on the face, especially around the eyebrows and in the folds on the cheeks.

Septra: *See* **Trimethoprim-sulfamethoxazole**.

Seroconversion: The process of developing an antibody to an infectious agent. In the case of HIV, it occurs shortly after primary infection.

Serologies: Blood tests that measures antibodies or antigens to look for evidence of a disease.

Sexually transmitted infections (STIs): Infections transmitted from person to person through sexual activity. Also called *sexually transmitted diseases (STDs)*.

Shingles (herpes zoster): A painful, blistering rash, usually occurring in a linear band on one side of the body, caused by reactivation of the chickenpox virus (varicella zoster virus, VZV).

"Shock and kill": An experimental cure strategy in which HIV-infected resting CD4 cells are first activated by latency-reversing agents, allowing the virus to be treated with antiretroviral therapy.

Side effects: Undesirable effects of a medication or treatment that are noticeable to the person being treated. *See also* **Toxicity**.

Sinus headache: A headache caused by congestion of the sinuses. *See also* **Sinusitis**.

Sinusitis: An infection of the sinuses—air spaces in the head connected to the nasal passages.

Social Security Disability Insurance (SSDI): A monthly Social Security benefit for disabled people who have worked in the past and have paid a minimum amount of Social Security taxes.

Sperm washing: A technique in which sperm are separated from semen to lower the risk of HIV transmission to a woman during conception.

Spinal tap (lumbar puncture): A procedure in which a needle is inserted into the back between the vertebrae to collect a sample of cerebrospinal fluid (CSF) to diagnose meningitis. (Not as bad as it sounds.)

SSDI: *See* **Social Security Disability Insurance**.

SSI: *See* **Supplemental Security Income**.

Statins: The common name for HMG CoA reductase inhibitors, drugs that lower cholesterol.

STIs: *See* **Sexually transmitted infections**.

Strain: In the case of HIV, a type of virus, as in drug-resistant strain.

Strep throat: The common term for streptococcal pharyngitis, a bacterial infection of the throat caused by group A beta-hemolytic *Streptococcus*.

Structured treatment interruption: An old term for an interruption in therapy that was approved by the provider.

Subcutaneous fat: Fat found under the skin.

Subtypes: In the case of HIV, groups of related viruses, also called "clades" or "sub-clades." Most HIV-positive people in the United States are infected with subtype B, but there are many other subtypes throughout the world.

Superinfection: Reinfection with a new strain of HIV in someone who has already been infected.

Supplemental Security Income (SSI): A federal cash assistance program designed to help the aged, blind, and disabled who have little or no income to pay for basic necessities.

Suppressor cell: *See* **CD8 cell**.

Symptomatic HIV infection: A stage of HIV infection in which people have symptoms caused by HIV, such as weight loss, diarrhea, or thrush, but have not yet developed an AIDS indicator condition.

Syndrome: A collection of signs or symptoms that frequently occur together but that may or may not be caused by a single disease. AIDS was referred to as a syndrome before its cause, HIV infection, had been discovered.

Syphilis: A sexually transmitted infection caused by *Treponema pallidum*, a bacterium, that can cause anal, genital, or mouth lesions (primary syphilis),

fever, rash, and hepatitis (secondary syphilis), or infection of the brain, spinal fluid, eyes, or ears (neurosyphilis). It can also be dormant, causing no symptoms (latent syphilis).

T

T-helper cell: *See* **CD4 cell**.

T-suppressor cells: *See* **CD8 cells**.

TB: *See* **Tuberculosis**.

Tdap: *See* **Tetanus toxoid**.

Tension headache: A headache caused by muscle tension.

Testosterone: The male sex hormone, which can be low in some HIV-positive men (*see* **Hypogonadism**).

Tetanus toxoid (dT or Tdap): A combination vaccine that should be received every 10 years for adults, regardless of HIV status. Tdap (a combination tetanus, diphtheria, pertussis vaccine) should be given once.

Therapeutic vaccine: A vaccine given to treat an existing infection by stimulating the immune system to fight it.

Thrombocytopenia: A disorder in which there is an abnormally low number of platelets in the blood.

Thrush: Oral candidiasis, a yeast infection involving the mouth presenting with white/yellow curd-like plaques on the palate, gums, or the back of the throat.

TMP-SMX: A combination of two antibiotic drugs used to treat a wide variety of bacterial infections. *See* **Trimethoprim-sulfamethoxazole**.

Toxicity: Damage to the body caused by a drug or other substance.

Toxoplasma: A parasite (*Toxoplasma gondii*) that causes brain lesions (encephalitis) in people with HIV infection.

Toxoplasmosis: Disease caused by the parasite, *Toxoplasma gondii*.

Transaminases (liver enzymes): Blood tests used to look for damage to the liver.

Transcription: The process of turning DNA into RNA.

Treatment interruption: Stopping antiretroviral therapy. No longer in vogue.

Triglycerides: Fats that are ingested in the form of vegetable oils and animal fats.

Trimethoprim-sulfamethoxazole (TMP-SMX, cotrimoxazole, *Bactrim*, *Septra*): An antibiotic used to treat or prevent PCP and to prevent toxoplasmosis.

Tropism assay: A blood test used to find out whether your virus enters the CD4 cell using the CCR5 coreceptor (R5 virus) or the CXCR4 coreceptor (X4 virus). This test is necessary before taking a CCR5 inhibitor, which should only be used with R5 virus.

Tuberculin skin test (TST): A skin test used to look for evidence of past exposure to *Mycobacterium tuberculosis*, the bacterium that causes tuberculosis. The most common form of TST is the PPD (purified protein derivative).

Tuberculosis (TB): A bacterial disease caused by *Mycobacterium tuberculosis*. TB most often causes lung disease but can affect any part of the body.

Typhoid vaccine: A vaccine to prevent typhoid fever, a bacterial infection of the blood caused by *Salmonella typhi*, sometimes acquired by travelers to developing countries.

U

Undetectable: A term used to describe a viral load that is too low to be measured by a viral load test. An undetectable viral load is below 20 with the most commonly used test.

Urinalysis: A standard lab test that looks for evidence of protein, sugar, blood, and infection in the urine.

V

Vaccine (vaccination): A substance that is given, usually by injection, but sometimes by mouth or by nasal spray, to stimulate the immune system to make antibodies against a bacterial or viral pathogen.

Vaginitis: Infection or inflammation of the vagina.

Valacyclovir: A drug used to treat herpes simplex and varicella zoster virus.

Varicella zoster virus: The virus that causes chickenpox (primary varicella) and shingles (herpes zoster).

Viral load (or plasma HIV RNA): A lab test that measures the amount of HIV virus in the plasma (blood), expressed as "copies per milliliter." The viral load predicts the rate of progression to AIDS. It is the most important test for measuring the effectiveness of ART and also helps determine the need for treatment.

Virions: Single virus particles.

Virus: A microscopic organism composed of genetic material (DNA or RNA) inside a protein coat.

Visceral fat: Fat present inside the abdomen, around the internal organs, rather than under the skin.

W

WB: *See* **Western blot**.

WBC: *See* **White blood cell**.

Western blot (WB): Traditionally, the confirmatory test used to

diagnosed HIV infection in people who tested positive for HIV antibodies by ELISA.

White blood cell (WBC): A type of blood cell that helps fight infection. CD4 cells are a type of lymphocyte, which is a type of white blood cell.

Wild-type virus: The strain of HIV that occurs "in the wild"—without the presence of antiretroviral drugs that could select for mutations. Generally a non-mutant, drug-sensitive virus.

Window period: The period between infection and formation of antibodies leading to a positive HIV test (serology).

X

X4 (or dual/mixed [D/M]) virus: HIV that enters the CD4 cell using the CXCR4 coreceptor. X4 virus cannot be treated with CCR5 inhibitors. (*See also* **Coreceptor**.)

Y

Yeast: A group of microorganisms that can sometimes cause human infections, ranging from minor (oral thrush, vaginitis) to severe (cryptococcal meningitis). All yeasts are fungi.

Yellow fever: A serious disease caused by yellow fever virus, which is transmitted by mosquitoes and sometimes acquired by travelers to parts of Africa or Latin America.

INDEX